Beasts OF THE Earth

Beasts
OF THE Earth

Animals, Humans, and Disease

E. Fuller Torrey, M.D.
Robert H. Yolken, M.D.

Rutgers University Press
New Brunswick, New Jersey, and London

Library of Congress Cataloging-in-Publication Data

Torrey, E. Fuller (Edwin Fuller), 1937–
    Beasts of the earth : animals, humans, and disease / E. Fuller Torrey, Robert H. Yolken.
        p.   ;   cm.
    Includes bibliographical references and index.
    ISBN 0-8135-3571-9 (hardcover : alk. paper)
    1. Zoonoses—Popular works.
    [DNLM: 1. Zoonoses—Popular Works.   2. Disease Outbreaks—Popular
Works.   3. Disease Transmission—Popular Works.   WC 950 T694b 2005]   I. Yolken,
Robert H.   II. Title.
    RA639.T676 2005
    616.9'59—dc22
                                                                    2004011751

A British Cataloging-in-Publication record for this book is available from the British Library

Copyright © 2005 by E. Fuller Torrey, M.D., and Robert H. Yolken, M.D.

Design by John Romer

Manufactured in the United States of America

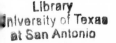

To our wives, Barbara and Faith

And God made the beasts of the earth according to their kinds and the cattle according to their kinds, and everything that creeps upon the ground according to its kind. And God saw that it was good.

GENESIS 1:24–25

And I saw, and behold, a pale horse, and its rider's name was Death, and Hades followed him; and they were given power over a fourth of the earth, to kill with sword and with famine and with pestilence and by wild beasts of the earth.

REVELATION 6:8

Contents

Acknowledgments

We are grateful to the following for helping to make this book possible:

Museo del Prado, Madrid, for permission to use a detail of Bosch's *Garden of Earthly Delights* for the cover.

Mr. Jordi Masia for arranging a visit to the remarkable Altamira caves, which helped us understand the relationship between Paleolithic people and animals.

Barbara Torrey and Dr. Robert Taylor for insightful and constructive comments on the manuscript.

Judy Miller for superb editing, organization, attention to detail, and the index.

Adi Hovav and Audra Wolfe at Rutgers University Press for their belief in the book during its conception and for midwifing its birth, Marilyn Campbell and Nicole Manganaro for excellent technical support, and Bobbe Needham for carefully copyediting the newborn manuscript.

Introduction

This book is about human infectious diseases and the microbes that cause them. As the recent resurgence of AIDS, tuberculosis, and influenza has shown, infections are still major causes of illness and death in our society. We are also discovering that infectious agents may play a role in many chronic ailments such as cancer, heart disease, and schizophrenia. The microbes that cause infectious diseases are thus very much part of our daily lives.

The vast majority of these microbes has been, and continues to be, transmitted to humans from other animals. A few diseases, heirloom infections such as those caused by herpes and hepatitis viruses, first infected our primate ancestors, and their microbes descended through early hominids to *Homo sapiens*. A large number of diseases, such as measles and tuberculosis, resulted from microbes transmitted to humans following the domestication of animals. Many other diseases, such as AIDS, SARS, mad cow disease, monkeypox, and bird flu have been transmitted from animals to humans in recent years as the relationship between animals and humans has changed. Each change in this relationship is accompanied by a risk of additional animal microbes being transmitted to humans.

We have become accustomed to thinking of animals as our friends, not as sources of human disease. Through the influence of Aesop, the Brothers Grimm, Beatrix Potter, and Walt Disney, it has become increasingly difficult to appreciate that the animal represented by Donald Duck was the origin of an influenza pandemic that killed twenty million people, that Mickey Mouse may be spreading deadly hantavirus, that Clarabelle Cow is the source of prions that cause mad cow disease, and that Pluto may be carrying leishmaniasis. We do not associate Bambi with Lyme disease, Big Bird with West Nile virus, Rocky Raccoon with rabies, or Garfield with toxoplasmosis. Even Barney, the dinosaur beloved of small children, is almost certainly a carrier of *Salmonella* bacteria, as all reptiles are.

In the past two hundred years, we have entered another period in which the relationship between animals and humans is changing in important ways. The changes include our personal relationship to animals as pets and ways of processing animals for our food supply. The present period of changing animal-human relationships may represent the most profound alteration in this relationship since animals were domesticated ten thousand years ago. One of the consequences of this changing relationship has been the emergence of new diseases that are transmitted to humans from animals.

Concurrent with the changing animal-human relationship have been changes in technology and in ways humans interact with each other. Changing sexual mores, the use of injections, increased urbanization, and increased access to air travel and other forms of transportation may all promote the spread of microbes from person to person. These changes magnify the effects of transmission of microbes from animals to humans, making it more likely that an infection of a single individual will become perpetuated as a chain of human infections.

It is important to appreciate the complexity of the animal-human relationship. On the one hand, animals have fulfilled many important human material and, as we have discovered more recently, psychological needs. On the other hand, animals have also been the source of many of the most important human diseases. These are the two sides of the beasts of the earth.

Beasts OF THE Earth

1

C H A P T E R

The Smallest Passengers on Noah's Ark

So, naturalists observe, a flea
Has smaller fleas that on him prey;
And these have smaller still to bite 'em;
And so proceed ad infinitum.

JONATHAN SWIFT, 1733

HUMAN diseases that are transmitted from animals are big news. Consider, for example, the following items reported in the United States during a single month, June 2003: 79 cases of human monkeypox, spread by pet prairie dogs; 7 cases of SARS (severe acute respiratory syndrome) among the 8,398 cases worldwide, spread by palm civets or other animals; the season's first human case of West Nile virus disease, spread from birds by mosquitoes; the season's first human case of Eastern equine encephalitis, spread from horses and other animals by mosquitoes; the first case of hantavirus infection, spread by mice and other rodents, in which two members of one family were infected; 2,820 new cases of Lyme disease, spread from deer by ticks, for the first half of the year; 19,482 new cases of AIDS, originally spread from primates, for the first half of the year; and a report of the first cow in North America infected with bovine spongiform encephalopathy (mad cow disease), which causes an almost invariably fatal disease when transmitted to humans.[1]

All of these are animal-associated diseases, caused by microbes, that may affect humans. In medical terms, they are called *zoonoses*. (Terms that may be new to readers are listed in the glossary.) Numerous news stories in recent years about such diseases have questioned whether zoonoses are becoming more numerous. The *Washington Post*, for example, published a front-page story on June 15, 2003, under the headline "Infections Now More Wide-spread: Animals Passing Them to Humans." Is there evidence to support an increasing incidence of animal-associated human diseases? As we shall see, there is.

In reading such news items, it is difficult to remember that humans are a relatively inconsequential part of the interaction between microbes and animals. Theologically, humans are said to be created in the image of God, but biologically we are merely one species in class Mammalia, phylum Craniata. There are 4,500 other species of mammals, encompassing everything from aardvarks, bats, cats, and rats to zebras, and including other primates. Anthropocentrally, we consider humans the most important animal species, yet all mammalian species combined constitute less than one-tenth of 1 percent of the estimated thirty million living animal species.[2] From the point of view of a microbe looking for an animal to parasitize, humans are at best an incidental hors d'oeuvre at a microbe's feast of life.

Where Do Microbes Come From?

The key to understanding animal-associated diseases is to understand microbes, referred to scientifically as *microorganisms*. They can be divided into microparasites, consisting of bacteria, viruses, fungi, and protozoa, and macroparasites, which include such organisms as helminths and tapeworms; macroparasites are comparatively unimportant as causes of serious human diseases. Prions, a newly discovered and poorly understood type of protein, will be discussed in chapter 8.

Stephen Jay Gould said bacteria are "the dominant form of life on Earth—and always have been, and probably always will be."[3] There are estimated to be between three hundred thousand and one million different species.[4] Ancestors of modern bacteria were the first form of life on earth, appearing approximately 3.5 billion years ago. (See the appendix for a time line of the evolution of life.) They are so primitive that bacterial cells do not even have nuclei; the genes simply float in the cells' cytoplasm and come together when the bacteria divide. Bacteria are also remarkably hardy, as was recently illustrated by the reported revival of bacteria that had lain quiescent in a salt crystal for 250 million years.[5]

Bacteria had existed for more than two billion years when other life forms came into being, and bacteria immediately colonized them. When fungi, plants, and animals emerged one billion years ago; when animal life diversified in the Cambrian explosion 570 million years ago; when land plants appeared 425 million years ago; when reptiles appeared 300 million years ago; when dinosaurs appeared and the continents drifted apart 200 million years ago; when mammals appeared 155 million years ago; when primates appeared 60 million years ago; when hominids separated from primates 6 million years ago; and when anatomically modern *Homo sapiens* emerged 130,000 years ago, bacteria were already ancient, adapted, and ready to take possession of these newly emerging life forms.

And take possession they did. The human mouth and large intestine each contain an estimated four hundred different *species* of bacteria. The total *number* of bacteria in the human large intestine has been estimated to be between one and ten trillion bacteria per milliliter.[6] Bacteria are also found in the human eye, ear, nose, stomach, small intestine, and genital tract and on the skin. It has been said that we have ten times as many bacteria as human cells in our bodies,[7] and that the bacteria account for a significant amount of the body weight.[8] Studies have shown that, although newborn infants are usually free from bacteria at birth, they are almost immediately colonized by bacteria and show the same distribution of normal flora as adults within a few weeks of birth.[9] All animals are similarly colonized, and all are carriers of bacteria.

Another measure of the importance of bacteria is that they have incorporated themselves into the genome of humans and other animals. This revelation was a surprising offshoot of the human genome sequencing project, in which it was reported "that between 113 and 223 genes have been transferred from bacteria to humans (or to one of our vertebrate ancestors) over the course of evolution."[10] Although subsequent analysis suggested that the actual number of transferred bacterial genes may be lower, that such transfers have occurred at all has led to a new appreciation of the importance of bacteria for humans and a reanalysis of the human relationship to bacterial ancestors. Many scientists suspect that the mitochondria found in all mammalian cells may also have originally come from bacteria that infected cells of our ancestors.

In contrast to those of bacteria, the origins and functions of viruses are poorly understood. A virus is not a living cell but merely one or two strands of DNA or RNA surrounded by a protein or lipoprotein coat, and it can reproduce itself only by getting into a living cell. Some researchers believe that viruses are degenerate forms of ancient bacteria, perhaps originally derived from plants. Others contend that viruses are pieces of animal genes that escaped from their cells, a kind of "rebel human DNA." A British astronomer has even suggested that viruses fell to earth from outer space.[11]

What is clear is that viruses are ubiquitous and have a complex and intimate relationship with humans and other animals. There are more than five thousand species of viruses known, and all of them, especially the RNA type, are unstable, undergo constant mutations, and are able to integrate their genetic material into other cells. Lewis Thomas, in his lyrical work *The Lives of a Cell*, described viruses as "more like mobile genes": "We live in a dancing matrix of viruses; they dart, rather like bees, from organism to organism, . . . tugging along pieces of this genome, strings of genes, . . . passing around heredity as though at a great party."[12] At least one type of RNA viruses, the endogenous (internal) retroviruses, not only can integrate themselves into the human genome but may also be passed on from generation to generation, just as inherited genes are (see chapter 2).

The third important type of microbe is protozoa. In popular parlance, bacteria, viruses, and protozoa together are called *germs*. Protozoa are also commonly referred to as *parasites*, although this is simply linguistic convention, since many bacteria and viruses are also parasites but are not referred to as such. Protozoa evolved from bacteria approximately two billion years ago. Like bacteria, protozoa are one-celled organisms, but unlike bacteria, they are more complex and have nuclei and other intracellular components such as mitochondria. Since they are very ancient, protozoa, like bacteria, also colonized other forms of life as these emerged, including humans and other animals.

That humans and other animals have been heavily colonized with bacteria, viruses, and protozoa since the beginning of our existence has been known for more than a century. American humorist Mark Twain, in an essay that he instructed not be published until after his death, wrote a satire about microbes on Noah's ark:

> Noah and his family . . . were saved, yes, but they were not comfortable, for they were full of microbes. Full to the eyebrows; fat with them, obese with them; distended like balloons. It was a disagreeable condition, but it could not be helped, because enough microbes had to be saved to supply the future races of men with desolating diseases, and there were but eight people on board to serve as hotels for them. . . . There were typhoid germs, and cholera germs, and hydrophobia germs, and lockjaw germs, and consumption germs, and black-plague germs, and some hundreds of other aristocrats, specially precious creations, golden bearers of God's love to man. . . . The great intestine was the favorite resort. There they gathered, by countless billions, and worked, and fed, and squirmed, and sang hymns of praise and thanksgiving; and at night when it was quiet you could hear the soft murmur of it. The large intestine was in effect their heaven.[13]

The fact that microbes cause human disease is thus not new. This discovery of the microbe-human disease relationship has been called "one of the greatest achievements of all time."[14] What *is* new is an increasing appreciation of the fact that many, if not most, of these microbes were originally transmitted to humans from other animals. And that this transmission is continuing to occur.

How Microbes Get Ahead in Life

All living organisms undergo continuous evolution, a process that is inherent in life itself. This is clearly visible for simpler forms of life, such as bacteria, viruses, and protozoa, which evolve more rapidly than complex forms of life such as mammals. But all living things evolve, as noted by Hans Zinsser in his classic *Rats, Lice, and History*: "Nothing in the world of living things is permanently fixed. Evolution is continuous, though its progress is so slow that the changes it produces can be perceived only in the determinable relationship of existing forms, and in their paleontological and embryological histories."[15]

One of the most common ways in which microbes evolve is by invading tissues of animals, including humans. In doing so, microbes are placed in a situation where they must evolve or die. Infectious diseases of animals and humans, therefore, are merely manifestations of microbes trying to get ahead in life. As Jared Diamond noted in *Guns, Germs, and Steel*: "Diseases represent evolution in progress, and microbes adapt by natural selection to new hosts and vectors. . . . In that new environment, a microbe must evolve new ways to live and to propagate itself."[16]

Humans and other animals, from a microbe's point of view, are merely vessels that are useful for reproducing and evolving. If a human or other animal becomes diseased as part of that process, the disease is incidental, that is, an epiphenomenon. It is not in the best interest of most bacteria, viruses, and protozoa to kill their host, because if they do so they may die as well. Arno Karlen, in *Man and Microbes*, described this process by noting that "the ultimate adjustment between host and parasite is not murder but mutuality. . . . Infectious disease, then, is not nature's tantrum against humanity. Often it is an argument in what becomes a long marriage."[17]

The outcome of this marriage, however, is not as clearly defined as it was once thought to be. For many years, it was believed that microbes and humans slowly learn to live with each other as microbes evolve toward a benign coexistence with their hosts. Thus, the bacterium that causes syphilis was thought to be extremely virulent when it initially spread among humans in the sixteenth century, then to have slowly become less virulent over the following three centuries. This reassuring view of microbial history has recently been challenged by Paul Ewald and others, who have questioned whether microbes do necessarily evolve toward long-term accommodation with their hosts. Under certain circumstances, Ewald argues: "Natural selection may . . . favor the evolution of extreme harmfulness if the exploitation that damages the host [i.e., disease] enhances the ability of the harmful variant to compete with a more benign pathogen."[18] The outcome of such a "marriage" may thus be the murder of one spouse by the other. In eschatological terms, this

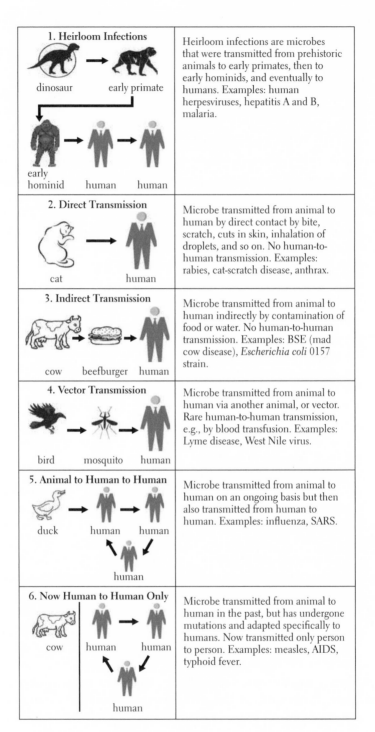

1. Heirloom Infections dinosaur → early primate early hominid → human → human	Heirloom infections are microbes that were transmitted from prehistoric animals to early primates, then to early hominids, and eventually to humans. Examples: human herpesviruses, hepatitis A and B, malaria.
2. Direct Transmission cat → human	Microbe transmitted from animal to human by direct contact by bite, scratch, cuts in skin, inhalation of droplets, and so on. No human-to-human transmission. Examples: rabies, cat-scratch disease, anthrax.
3. Indirect Transmission cow → beefburger → human	Microbe transmitted from animal to human indirectly by contamination of food or water. No human-to-human transmission. Examples: BSE (mad cow disease), *Escherichia coli* 0157 strain.
4. Vector Transmission bird → mosquito → human	Microbe transmitted from animal to human via another animal, or vector. Rare human-to-human transmission, e.g., by blood transfusion. Examples: Lyme disease, West Nile virus.
5. Animal to Human to Human duck → human → human → human	Microbe transmitted from animal to human on an ongoing basis but then also transmitted from human to human. Examples: influenza, SARS.
6. Now Human to Human Only cow | human → human → human	Microbe transmitted from animal to human in the past, but has undergone mutations and adapted specifically to humans. Now transmitted only person to person. Examples: measles, AIDS, typhoid fever.

FIGURE 1-1: Types of Animal-to-Human Transmission of Microbes

view argues that a microbe such as HIV or SARS virus may be truly capable of eradicating the human race.

Microbes are remarkably resourceful in finding ways to move from animals to humans. As shown in figure 1.1, the transmission of microbes from animals to humans may occur in a variety of ways. Some transmissions from early animals to hominids took place in the distant past, before *Homo sapiens* had even evolved, and then the microbes were passed down from hominids to humans (panel 1); these are called *heirloom infections* (see chapter 2). Direct transmission occurs when animals pass microbes directly to humans (panel 2), such as when a cat scratches a human, causing cat-scratch disease; when a dog bites a human, causing rabies; or when a person inhales aerosolized mouse droppings and gets hantavirus infection. Indirect transmission occurs when there is an intermediary between the animals and the humans (panel 3), such as when a cow becomes infected with bovine spongiform encephalopathy (mad cow disease) and after death passes the prion to humans by way of beef-burgers, or when an infected cow transmits the toxic strain of *Escherichia coli* bacteria by way of contaminated food or water. Another mode of transmission is when the microbe hitchhikes on another animal, called a *vector*, such as a mosquito, tick, flea, or fly (panel 4). Examples of this include the West Nile virus, which uses mosquitoes to move from birds to humans; the bacteria that causes Lyme disease, which uses ticks to move from deer to humans; and the plague bacteria, which uses fleas to move from rats to humans. Whatever mode of transportation the microbe chooses, the objective is always the same: Be fruitful and multiply.

When animal microbes are transmitted to humans for the first time, most of the microbes either die or pass harmlessly through our bodies without our being aware of them. A few microbes cause infections in humans that may result in symptoms of illness or even in death. In most such cases, the microbe cannot be passed from human to human, as illustrated in the examples in panels 2, 3, and 4 in figure 1.1. Occasionally, however, the microbe adapts itself to humans, usually by undergoing minor changes in its genetic makeup called *mutations*, and is then able to spread from human to human (panel 5). Transmission of the microbe from animal to human continues to take place, but human-to-human transmission also occurs; influenza and SARS are examples.

Finally, in a few cases, after the microbe has been adapted to humans for a long period of time, it changes its genetic makeup so much that it is no longer transmitted from animals to humans but only from humans to humans (panel 6). Examples are measles, which originally was transmitted to humans from cattle; AIDS, which was originally transmitted from primates; and typhoid fever, which was originally transmitted from birds. This type of animal-to-human transmission differs from an heirloom infection in that the original transmission occurred after *Homo sapiens* had evolved, that is, within the past 130,000 years.

Being resourceful, many microbes have developed multiple modes of transmission. The protozoa that causes sleeping sickness (trypanosomiasis), for example, is transmitted among horses as a venereal disease, among humans by using flies as a vector, and among rats by using fleas as a vector.[19] In the course of evolving, microbes often develop new methods of moving from one animal to another. A recent example of this is the virus that causes SARS, which apparently found ways to move from palm civets or other animals to humans and then from human to human.

All microbes are continuously trying to spread themselves, crossing both geographic and species barriers. Humans are therefore subjected to a continuing barrage of bacteria, viruses, and protozoa coming from other animals. Given this continuous exposure, it is remarkable that we do not suffer more than we do from animal-associated diseases.

There are three major determinants that influence the outcome of encounters between a microbe and a potentially new host such as a human: genes, the immune system, and the virulence of the microbe. Genetic expression varies from person to person and plays an important role in determining whether or not a microbe will cause illness. For example, half the people in the world are infected with the bacteria *Helicobacter pylori*. However, the bacteria causes disease, such as gastric ulcers or stomach cancer, in fewer than one in five of the *Helicobacter* carriers. One factor that determines whether the bacteria will cause disease is whether the person has certain genes (specifically the babA2, cagA, or vacA genotypes).[20] Having these genes does not guarantee that *Helicobacter* will cause disease, but it increases the odds that it will. Such genes are called *predisposing genes*, and there are probably dozens, or even hundreds, of such genes for all human diseases that are caused by microbes.

Another example is *Mycobacterium tuberculosis*, which infects large numbers of individuals. However, only one out of ten people infected with this bacteria develops tuberculosis. It is now known that carrying certain genes, such as NRAMP-1 or a specific type of vitamin D receptor (VDR) gene, predisposes a person to develop clinical tuberculosis.[21]

Genes may predispose individuals to diseases caused by microbes, but they may also be protective. The best-known example of this is the protection provided against malaria by the gene associated with sickle-cell disease. Individuals who carry the sickle hemoglobin gene are more resistant to infection by *Plasmodium falciparum*, protozoa that cause the most severe form of malaria. Another example of a protective gene is PTR-1, a gene that limits the damage induced by protozoa that causes leishmaniasis, a disease spread by dogs (see chapter 7).[22]

Many of the genes that predispose or protect an individual in encounters with microbes do so by affecting the person's immune system, the second determinant of the outcome. This is an extraordinarily complex system that consists of lymphocytes and other white blood cells, cytokines, and antibodies against microbes. Anything that weakens the immune system makes a person more susceptible to infection; conversely, anything that strengthens the system makes a person more resistant. The former is illustrated by individuals with AIDS who become increasingly susceptible to all infections as their lymphocytes become fewer in number.

The third major determinant that influences the outcome of encounters between microbes and potentially new hosts is the strength, or virulence, of the microbe. Bacteria, viruses, and protozoa all have strains that are more lethal or less lethal; this variation is commonly called *virulence*. A well-known example of this is the influenza virus: Some strains cause only a mild illness; other strains, such as the one that caused the 1918 influenza pandemic, are highly lethal.

Occasionally, different kinds of microbes join forces to cause disease. In mice, for example, the mouse hepatitis virus is harmless by itself, and the protozoan *Eperythrozoon coccoides* is harmless by itself, but when they infect mice together, the mice develop severe hepatitis and die.[23] Such co-infections are also known to occur in humans; for example, the hepatitis D virus is harmless by itself but can cause severe disease when the person is also infected with the hepatitis B virus.

Encounters between microbes and their potential hosts thus resemble battle scenes from Star Wars. The outcome of such battles depends in part on the numbers and strength (virulence) of the invading microbes and in part on the strength of the defensive forces (genes that afford resistance) and its special weapons (the immune system). Traitors within the defensive forces (predisposing genes) may tip the scales in favor of the invaders. Cells of the immune system may also act as Trojan horses, carrying microbes to previously uninfected parts of the body. These battles occur continuously in humans and in all other animals.

As humans, it is understandable that we focus attention on the effects of microbes on ourselves. However, it is important to keep in mind that microbes similarly affect all other animal species, sometimes with catastrophic results. An example was the rinderpest virus epidemic among African animals in the closing years of the nineteenth century. The virus, which was endemic among cattle in India, was brought to Africa for the first time in 1889, when the Italian army imported cattle from India to feed its troops in Ethiopia and Somalia. Rinderpest quickly infected African domestic cattle, sweeping across the continent within seven years and virtually wiping them out in many areas.

Since cattle were the main source of food for African groups such as the Masai, widespread human famine followed. As one Masai man described the epidemic, the corpses of cattle and people were "so many and so close together that the vultures had forgotten how to fly."[24] The rinderpest epidemic also spread to wild animals related to cattle, causing especially widespread mortality among buffalo, wildebeests, giraffes, bushpigs, eland, and kudu.

The African rinderpest epidemic was an example of the spread of a microbe from one animal to another of the same species (Indian to African cattle) and to other species in the same animal order (cattle, buffalo, wildebeests, etc., all of which are artiodactyls). A more recent example of such an epidemic was the death of at least 30 percent of North Sea grey seals by the phocine distemper virus. This virus had been endemic among harp seals in the Arctic region, but the harp seals migrated to the North Sea after commercial overfishing depleted Arctic fish stocks.[25]

Less commonly, microbes may spread from one species to a species in a different animal order. An example of this was the spread to seals of canine distemper virus, which was endemic among dogs. Dogs are members of the carnivore order of mammals, while seals are members of the pinniped order. The canine distemper virus is thought to have been introduced to Antarctic seals by contact with infected sled dogs used on Antarctic explorations.[26] Canine distemper virus also caused a devastating epidemic among seals in the Caspian Sea. The origin of the virus became clear when it was learned that people who lived nearby had thrown dogs that had died from a local outbreak of canine distemper into the sea, where they were eaten by the seals.[27] Another carnivore-to-pinniped transmission (cat to sea otter) recently occurred along the northern California coast. The protozoan *Toxoplasma gondii*, excreted by cats, washed into the sea with groundwater runoff from streams that drained an area with large numbers of cats, with the resultant death of many sea otters.[28]

As a general rule, then, when microbes spread, they are most likely to spread to other members of the same species or to members of closely related species. Thus, humans are most likely to become infected by microbes coming from other humans, then by microbes coming from other primates, then by microbes coming from other mammals, and so on. The more closely related the animals, the more likely it is that microbes will be exchanged between them.

Also, as interested as we are as humans in the transmission of microbes from other animals to ourselves, we need to keep in mind that microbes move freely in both directions. Humans have inadvertently transmitted to primates human microbes that cause polio, tuberculosis, malaria, and influenza, and probably pneumonia, meningitis, and measles.[29] There are also documented instances of the spread of antibiotic-resistant staphylococcus bacteria from humans to cats, dogs, and horses, causing infections in these animals.[30]

At the same time that existing microbes are spreading among related and unrelated animal species, new microbes continue to evolve. This occurs when the genetic structure of existing microbes undergoes slight modifications. A recent example of this was mutations of the feline panleukopenia virus (FPV), a cat virus first described in the early twentieth century. In the 1940s, a new viral disease of minks was noted; the cause was subsequently found to be mink parvovirus (MPV), which was a mutation of FPV. Then, in the 1970s, a new disease of domestic dogs was described, and its causative agent, named canine parvovirus (CPV), was also shown to be a mutation of FPV. Genetic mapping studies have shown that FPV, MPV, and CPV differ by changes in only a few nucleotides.[31] The FPV virus had been evolving, spreading by mutations from one species of animal to another and causing new diseases.

How Many Human Infections Come from Animals?

How many human infections are caused by microbes that spread from other animals? Researchers at the University of Edinburgh recently compiled a list of 1,415 microbes known to cause diseases in humans. Of these, 868, or 61 percent, are known to be currently transmitted from other animals to humans.[32] Significantly, this list did not include microbes that were transmitted from other animals to humans in the recent past, such as the HIV virus from chimpanzees, which probably occurred in the last fifty years, or in the more distant past, such as the measles virus from cows, which occurred approximately ten thousand years ago. If all examples of past animal-to-human microbe transmissions are included in the list, it seems likely that at least three-quarters of all human infections are caused by microbes that originally came from animals. Most of the other one-quarter of human infections are almost certainly heirloom infections, transmitted from animals to hominids before modern humans evolved.

From which animals do microbes that cause human diseases come? According to the Scottish researchers, the largest number come from dogs and cats (carnivores, 43 percent) and from domestic livestock, primarily horses, cattle, sheep, goats, and pigs (ungulates, 39 percent). Additional microbes that cause human diseases come from rodents (23 percent), other primates (13 percent), birds (10 percent), marine mammals (5 percent), and bats (2 percent). The total adds up to more than 100 percent because some microbes may be transmitted to humans from more than one animal; rabies, for example, may come from dogs, cats, raccoons, and bats. In fact, this study concluded that "over a quarter of pathogens of humans and domestic mammals have a very broad host range and are capable of infecting human, domestic and wildlife hosts."[33]

In addition to asking how many infectious diseases are caused by microbes transmitted from animals, researchers have also asked how many of the *emerging* human infectious diseases are caused by microbes transmitted from animals. By "emerging," researchers mean diseases caused by microbes "that have appeared in a human population for the first time, or have occurred previously but are increasing in incidence or expanding into areas where they had not . . . been reported" in the past twenty years.[34] SARS and avian influenza (bird flu) are examples of such emerging diseases. This question has been raised because of an increasingly broad consensus among specialists in infectious diseases that "in the past few years, emergent disease episodes have increased in the United States and globally. . . . Nearly all these emergent disease episodes have involved zoonotic infectious agents."[35]

In an attempt to quantify emergent diseases, the Scottish researchers made a list of 175 microbes that are known to cause emerging infectious diseases in humans. Of these, 132, or 75 percent, are transmitted from animals.[36] Viruses account for 44 percent of these animal-associated emergent human infections, bacteria for 30 percent, protozoa for 11 percent, and helminths and fungi together for the remaining 15 percent. RNA viruses are especially prominent, since their mutation rate is significantly higher than that of other microbes, and they can therefore adapt more quickly to new hosts.[37] The importance of animal-associated microbes as the cause of emerging human diseases has thus been clearly established. In 2004, the director of the Centers for Disease Control and Prevention, Dr. Julie Gerberding, noted that "11 of the last 12 emerging infectious diseases that we're aware of in the world, that have had human health consequences, have probably arisen from animal sources."[38] As summarized by a report from the Institute of Medicine: "The significance of zoonoses in the emergence of human infections cannot be overstated."[39]

The available data on zoonoses probably underestimate their contribution to human diseases. One reason for this is "the inherent bias of humans in studying themselves in preference to other species," according to the Scottish research group that catalogued these diseases.[40] Much more is known about microbes that affect humans than about those that affect other animals; as the latter become better known, the animal origins of additional human diseases likely will become evident.

Knowledge about the origins of microbes in general will very probably increase rapidly in the coming years. We now have the ability to determine the nucleic acid sequences of viruses, bacteria, and protozoa and to compare those sequences with the sequences of related microbes. This enables researchers to create phylogenetic trees for microbes, arranging the microbes' ancestors just as is done for human family trees. As a general rule, the greater the difference in the nucleic acid sequence between two related microbes, the longer ago they diverged from a common ancestor. Various "molecular clocks" are used to estimate that time interval.[41]

Finally, in the ongoing war between microbes and humans, microbes have a definite advantage. In any war, the winner's victory partly depends on its having been able to perceive its enemy's defenses, then adapting its forces to exploit weaknesses in those defenses. Bacteria and viruses can reproduce and create a new generation of themselves in a few minutes, protozoa, in a few days. Humans, by contrast, need twenty years to reproduce and create a new generation. If speed of evolution and adaptability is to be the deciding factor in the ongoing war between microbes and humans, the future of the human race is not bright. Clearly, we need to continue developing other weapons in the human arsenal, including anti-infective drugs, vaccines, and measures to prevent infections, if we are to survive. As noted by Richard Krause, former director of the National Institute of Allergy and Infectious Diseases, microbes were on earth for more than two billion years before humans arrived, "and it is likely that they will be here 2 billion years after we depart."[42]

2

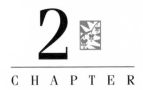

CHAPTER

Heirloom Infections

Microbes before the Advent of Humans

> *Belief in a golden age has provided mankind with solace in times of despair. . . . The very belief in its existence implies the conviction that perfect health and happiness are birthrights of men. Yet, in reality, complete freedom from disease and from struggle is almost incompatible with the process of living.*
>
> RENE DUBOS, *Mirage of Health*

IF THERE ever was a Garden of Eden, it certainly was not free from disease. Adam may have been carrying the herpesviruses that cause cold sores and shingles, and Eve could have had hepatitis B. Mosquitoes in the garden may have been carrying the microbes that cause malaria and yellow fever. And the serpent that proffered Eve the forbidden fruit was almost certainly carrying *Salmonella* bacteria, as reptiles had been doing for millions of years. One hopes that Eve washed the apple before eating it and offering it to Adam.

Given that bacteria, viruses, and protozoa had existed for millions of years before animals evolved, it is not surprising that the earliest known animals were infected with microbes. Evidence of staphylococcus infection of a reptile bone has been dated to approximately two hundred million years ago, a viral infection in a bird fossil to ninety million years ago, and a bacterial abscess in a dinosaur jaw to at least seventy-five million years ago.[1] As mammals evolved from reptiles, primates from mammals, hominids from primates, and *Homo sapiens* from hominids, all were exposed to the existing bacteria, viruses, and protozoa.

Often, microbes that infected earlier species of animals were passed along to later species as the later species evolved. Thus, as hominids evolved from primates, they carried with them bacteria, viruses, and protozoa that had infected primates. These infections have been called *heirloom infections*, since they are similar to possessions from our parents and grandparents that many of us carry with us from generation to generation.[2]

Most microbes that cause heirloom infections are harmless, living unobtrusively on our skin or in our intestines for our entire lives. Such microbes are called *commensals*, and many are useful to us, such as intestinal bacteria that help us digest food. Commensal microbes rarely cause disease except when their distribution changes or when the host's defense mechanisms change. Examples of such circumstances are treatment with antibiotics, which changes the distribution of microbes, or AIDS, in which the body's immune defenses are markedly reduced. In many cases, if we leave human heirloom infections alone, they will leave us alone.

Human heirloom infections include protozoa commonly found in human intestines. One study reported that among twelve human intestinal protozoa, eleven are also found in the intestines of monkeys.[3] Similarly, the protozoa *Trichomonas vaginalis*, which may cause a mild vaginal infection in women, has been isolated from both wild and captive monkeys, in which the symptoms are also mild.[4]

The consequences of having inherited microbes from our ancestors are also illustrated by the appearance of similar microbes in humans everywhere on earth. This is especially true of harmless commensal microbes; as noted by one researcher: "Isolated human tribes have the same commensals as those living in well populated areas."[5] Thus, the types of bacteria in the noses of humans who live in remote villages in Papua New Guinea are remarkably similar to the microbes found in the noses of people who live in New York and Paris.

Herpes and Hepatitis Viruses

Although most human heirloom infections are harmless, some may cause disease. Examples are infections with human herpesviruses and some of the viruses that cause hepatitis.

All members of the herpesvirus family are thought to have evolved from a common herpesvirus ancestor that originated approximately 400 million years ago. This ancestor virus split into two ancestral lines. One of these evolved into the herpesviruses that today infect fish (e.g., channel catfish virus) and amphibians such as frogs (e.g., ranid herpesvirus 1). When birds and mammals evolved, the other ancestor herpesvirus split approximately 180 million years ago into three main families, labeled alpha, beta, and gamma. These families in turn further divided, so that, for example, approximately 8 million years ago, herpes simplex virus 2, which is a common cause of genital infections, split off from herpes simplex virus 1, which may cause cold sores. As described by researchers: "The overall scheme of herpesvirus evolution . . . places the development of herpesviruses in much the same timeframe as that of the vertebrates."[6] The simultaneous evolution of microbes such as viruses with other life forms is referred to as *coevolution*, indicating that the two evolved together. Since all forms of life are continuously evolving, coevolution of microbes and animals is also continuous in what is essentially a phylogenetic pas de deux. It is a Darwinian dance that is never ending.

Today, there are eight known human herpesviruses, and it is likely that there are additional, undiscovered ones. They are divided into the alpha, beta, and gamma families that were established 180 million years ago. Since herpesviruses have been coevolving with other mammals and birds, herpesviruses also infect other species. Table 2.1 lists the known human herpesviruses with the diseases caused by them; it also includes selected examples of herpesviruses that occur in other animals.

Human herpesviruses have some common characteristics. All of them, for example, establish lifetime infections in their hosts. They may remain quietly latent for long periods of time, causing no symptoms, and then suddenly flare up, as occurs with infections of herpes simplex viruses 1 and 2 or varicella-zoster virus. The herpesviruses are also noteworthy for the variety of illnesses they may cause in a single animal species. In humans, for example, they may cause cold sores, childhood rashes, mononucleosis, and various forms of cancer.

Members of each family of herpesviruses are more closely related to each other than to members of another family; thus, herpes simplex virus 1 of humans is more closely related to canine herpesvirus 1 of dogs or feline herpesvirus 1 of cats than it is to human cytomegalovirus or Epstein-Barr virus. As noted in chapter 1, the more closely related the animal species, the more likely it is that a virus from one species will be transmitted to another species. This is illustrated by the herpes B virus of macaque monkeys. In monkeys, the herpes B virus is transmitted either sexually or orally and produces a mild infection similar to that produced by herpes simplex 1 and 2 in humans. However, when humans are bitten by monkeys infected with the herpes B virus, the virus may be transmitted to humans, causing a severe, and often fatal, infection of the brain (encephalitis). Transmission of herpesviruses from dogs, cats, or other animals more distantly related to humans is not known to occur.

Another important principle illustrated by herpesviruses is that, even though the heirloom infections they cause have existed in humans since

TABLE 2.1. Herpesviruses of Humans and Other Animals

Type of Virus	Animals Infected	Symptoms
Alpha herpesviruses		
*Herpes simplex virus 1**	Humans	Cold sores, occasional brain infections
Herpes simplex virus 2	Humans	Genital infections, infections of newborns
Varicella-zoster virus	Humans	Chickenpox (varicella), shingles (herpes zoster)
Herpes B virus	Monkeys	
Simian agent 8	Baboons	
Spider-monkey herpesvirus	Monkeys	
Canine herpesvirus 1	Dogs	
Feline herpesvirus 1	Cats	
Equine herpesvirus 1	Horses	
Equine herpesvirus 4	Horses	
Bovine herpesvirus 1	Cattle	
Marek's disease virus	Birds	
Infectious laryngotracheitis virus	Birds	
Beta herpesviruses		
Human cytomegalovirus	Humans	Usually asymptomatic but can cause congenital infections in fetus and immune-compromised individual
Human herpesvirus 6	Humans	Childhood rash (exanthem subitum)
Human herpesvirus 7	Humans	No disease yet known
Murine cytomegalovirus	Mice	

(*continued*)

TABLE 2.1. (*continued*)

Type of Virus	Animals Infected	Symptoms
Gamma herpesviruses		
Epstein-Barr virus	Humans	Mononucleosis, Burkitt's lymphoma, nasopharyngeal carcinoma
Human herpesvirus 8	Humans	Kaposi's sarcoma, often associated with HIV infection
Herpesvirus saimiri	Monkeys	
Equine herpesvirus 2	Horses	
Murine herpesvirus 68	Mice	

*Human viruses appear in italics.

SOURCE: Adapted from D. J. McGeoch, S. Cook, A. Dolan et al., "Molecular Phylogeny and Evolutionary Timescale for the Family of Mammalian Herpesviruses," *Journal of Molecular Biology* 247 (1995): 443–458.

Homo sapiens evolved, these infections may change as humans change. For example, herpes simplex virus 2, which is transmitted sexually, has markedly increased in incidence in recent years as human sexual practices have changed. Similarly, human herpesvirus 8 was unknown until the AIDS epidemic but has been recognized as the cause of Kaposi's sarcoma, a form of cancer that occurs with greatly increased frequency when a person's immune system is markedly weakened.

Other examples of human heirloom infections are hepatitis A and hepatitis B viruses. (Hepatitis C is almost certainly also an heirloom infection, but its origin has not been studied as extensively.) Hepatitis A is a common cause of acute human hepatitis in the United States. The virus is usually spread by person-to-person contact or by contaminated food or water, especially in places where sanitary conditions are poor.

Outbreaks of hepatitis A have also occurred among animal handlers who work closely with chimpanzees and other primates. We therefore know that hepatitis A can spread from primates to humans, and it is suspected that it can also spread from humans to primates. Recent analyses of hepatitis A strains in primates and humans have shown that they are closely related, suggesting a common viral ancestor.[7]

Hepatitis B is caused by a virus unrelated to the virus that causes hepatitis A. It affects 5 percent of the human population and causes cirrhosis and cancer of the liver, resulting in approximately one million deaths per year worldwide. It is transmitted by sexual contact, the sharing of needles, and blood transfusions, and from mothers to infants via blood contact during the delivery process.

The family to which the hepatitis B virus belongs, hepadnaviruses, includes related viruses that affect birds, squirrels, woodchucks, and several primates. The virus most closely related to the human hepatitis B virus is found in woolly monkeys, suggesting that the human and primate viruses may have descended from a common ancestor.[8] Hepatitis B virus can be transmitted experimentally from humans to other primates such as chimpanzees, but it is not known whether transmission can also occur from primates to humans.

Malaria and Yellow Fever

Malaria is a classic heirloom infection that has affected primates since they evolved approximately sixty million years ago. It causes approximately two million human deaths each year worldwide, half of them of children under five. But its devastation is even broader, because millions of other people with chronic malaria suffer from periodic fevers and severe anemia, with resulting lack of energy.

Malaria has also changed the course of history. According to Richard Fiennes, an expert in tropical diseases: "The results of malarial infection on the evolution and history of civilized man have been incalculable." Fiennes claims that malaria "may well have been a major cause of the decline and fall of the Greek and Roman empires" and "has been responsible for the devitalization of whole populations."[9] Malaria is thus one of the oldest and one of the deadliest human diseases.

Four species of *Plasmodium* protozoa (malaria parasites)—*vivax, ovale, malariae,* and *falciparum*—infect humans, and at least twenty-five other species infect reptiles, birds, rodents, and other mammals. A major reason these protozoa have been so successful is that they learned to use blood-sucking mosquitoes as vectors to move from host to host. This was much more efficient than traveling on their own, and over millions of years these protozoa developed a complex life cycle in which one part of their reproductive stage occurs in mosquitoes.

The protozoa that cause human malaria descended from primates through various hominids to *Homo sapiens. Vivax, ovale,* and *malariae* separated from related primate protozoa approximately twenty-five to thirty million years ago, whereas *falciparum* separated from a chimpanzee protozoan five to ten million years ago.[10]

Since that time, the *Plasmodium* species that infect humans have changed genetically so that, with the possible exception of *malariae*, they can no longer naturally infect other primates. On the other hand, three *Plasmodium* species found in primates have, on rare occasions, been naturally transmitted by mosquitoes from primates to humans.[11] Thus, malaria is both an heirloom infection, transmitted millions of years ago from primates to hominids and eventually to humans, and also a contemporary although rare zoonosis still being transmitted from primates to humans.

Yellow fever, like malaria, is both an heirloom infection and an ongoing zoonosis. In humans, it varies from being a mild febrile illness to being a severe illness with high fever, internal hemorrhaging, jaundice, kidney failure, and death. It was brought to the Americas with African slaves. In Philadelphia in 1793, a yellow-fever epidemic killed 10 percent of the population and shut down the U.S. government, which was temporarily housed in that city. In Memphis in 1878, it halved the population and caused twenty thousand deaths in the Mississippi Valley.[12]

Yellow fever has often altered the course of history. In Haiti, for example, the 1801 uprising of African slaves was successful because yellow fever killed twenty-seven thousand French troops while leaving untouched the African-born slaves, who were relatively immune because of their exposure earlier in life. Napoleon, discouraged by the loss of his Haitian colony, gave up his American ambitions and sold his remaining territory, the Louisiana Purchase. The combination of yellow fever and malaria also affected the colonization of Africa, since "about half of the European missionaries died [from these diseases] during their first year in Africa. . . . For this reason, they often shipped their gear [to Africa] in a coffin."[13] Yellow fever was also a major reason for the failure of the French to build a canal between the Atlantic and the Pacific at the Isthmus of Panama in the nineteenth century. The control of the disease through control of the mosquitoes was one reason for the eventual success of the U.S. builders of the canal in the early part of the twentieth century.

The yellow-fever virus has apparently been endemic in African monkeys for millions of years and causes no apparent disease in them. Like the malaria protozoa, the yellow-fever virus evolved ways of using mosquitoes as vectors to move from host to host. And as with malaria, control of the disease is through eradication of the mosquitoes that carry it.

Urban yellow fever is an heirloom infection in that monkeys are no longer involved in its transmission. The virus simply moves from human to human, carried by mosquitoes that breed in still water. Jungle yellow fever, by contrast, involves transmission from monkeys to humans and primarily affects individuals who live near forested areas.

Endogenous Retroviruses

A special type of heirloom infection involves endogenous retroviruses. These are retroviruses in the same large family as HIV, the virus that causes AIDS, and HTLV, a virus that causes a type of leukemia and a neurological disorder. Endogenous retroviruses are able to integrate themselves into the sperm and egg cells and thus be passed down from generation to generation. Such integrations have occurred many times in the history of *Homo sapiens* and our progenitors. One period of integration was approximately thirty-five million years ago, after New World monkeys split off from the other primates but before *Homo sapiens* became distinguished from other primates. It was during this period that the integration of a virus known as Human Endogenous Retrovirus W (Herv-W) took place. We know this because humans share a number of Herv-W genetic sequences with all the Old World primates, including rhesus monkeys, gibbons, apes, and chimpanzees, but not with New World monkeys such as macaques or squirrel monkeys.

Integrations of other retroviruses into the human genome have occurred at more recent times in primate evolution. One type of retrovirus has been found in humans, chimpanzees, and gorillas but not in orangutans and gibbons, suggesting that this integration occurred after the split of these species approximately ten million years ago. Other integrations appear to have occurred even more recently. One type of retrovirus, known as Herv-K, is found mostly in humans. One strain of Herv-K occurs in some humans but not others, indicating that the original attack of this retrovirus and its integration into the genome occurred after the separation of different groups of *Homo sapiens* approximately one hundred thousand years ago.

Interestingly, in all of these cases the infectious retroviruses that originally attacked our ancestors appear to have disappeared from the face of the earth. Such viruses live on only in our genes and in the genes of our primate cousins. It is possible that the process is still going on, and that we will genetically pass on to future generations the retroviruses that are currently infecting human populations, such as HIV, HTLV-1, and HTLV-2.

The persistence of these retroviruses in the primate genome—for millions of years, in some cases—has led scientists to ask whether the viruses have persisted because they offer some protective advantage. In fact, some of the retroviruses have been commandeered by the human genome to perform important functions; for example, one of the retrovirus proteins appears to be important in the formation of the human placenta. Other parts of these retroviruses are used to control the expression of primate genes, particularly those involved in the regulation of the immune response to microbes. This apparently allows humans and other primates, which have relatively slow rates of procreation, to respond more rapidly to environmental changes. For example, it is possible that the presence of these retroviruses in our genomes protects us from infection with many other retroviruses to which we are exposed. This may be why we do not apparently become infected with retroviruses from monkeys, cats, mice, rats, chickens, and many other animals with which we are in contact. However, the recent emergence of HIV and HTLV-1 indicates that such protection is not total.

The aberrant expression of endogenous retroviruses in our genome has been suspected, but not proven, to be associated with a number of human diseases, including multiple sclerosis, schizophrenia, and systemic lupus, and with problems during pregnancy, including preeclampsia. It thus may be that the protection these endogenous retroviral heirloom infections offer us comes at a price. Our ability to understand and control the expression of these heirloom infections would represent a major accomplishment in the field of human health.

Hominids, then, have been continuously infected with microbes ever since they began evolving from their primate ancestors. Many of these microbes had also infected the mammalian ancestors of primates and even the premammalian ancestors, such as reptiles and birds. Human diseases such as herpes infections, hepatitis A and B, malaria, yellow fever, and endogenous retroviral infections are thus heirloom infections, part of our birthright as humans.

Most worrisome about heirloom infections is what we do not know. Most microbes that are part of the human legacy are harmless, and we live with them in negotiated peace. The emergence of human herpesvirus 8 as a cause of Kaposi's sarcoma in individuals with AIDS, when the immune system has been devastated, has given us pause. How many other unknown microbes that we carry as our heritage may do harm under changing biological circumstances?

3

CHAPTER

Humans as Hunters

Animal Origins of Bioterrorism

Unlike the remaining living primates, man evolved as a carnivorous pred-
ator dependent on his mental and physical prowess to kill other animals
for food. This entailed the development of complicated social relationships
between the hunters, their prey, and competing predators.

JULIET CLUTTON-BROCK, *Domestic Animals from Early Times*

EARLY hominids had little contact with animals other than themselves.
The ancestors of *Homo sapiens*, after breaking away from other African
apes approximately six million years ago, subsisted on a diet mostly of insects,
fruits, and leaves and apparently did little hunting of animals.

The best measure of what early hominids ate is probably what modern
chimpanzees eat. Jane Goodall, who studied these animals in Tanzania, observed them eating more than fifty types of fruit, thirty types of leaves and leaf
buds, blossoms, seeds, bark, nuts, ants, termites, caterpillars, honey, and larval
grubs of bees, wasps, and beetles. Chimpanzees occasionally also eat birds'
eggs and meat from other animals, including baboons, monkeys, and young
bushbucks or bushpigs, but these are not mainstays of their diet. Goodall estimated that one chimpanzee eats the equivalent of approximately one-half
a prey animal in a one-year period, and during ten years of observation, she
observed chimpanzees killing other animals only twice.[1]

Even when *Australopithecus afarensis* walked upright on the African
plains approximately three million years ago, the dietary practices of early
hominids had not changed much. An analysis of the teeth of "Lucy," the best-
studied member of this group, suggests she ate fruit "in quantities when it was
in season, . . . a great many berries and seeds and roots and tubers, and a good

deal of dirt and sand along with these things."[2] These hominids undoubtedly supplemented their diet with small animals when they could catch them, but meat was not a major part of their diet.

It was not until approximately one million years ago that human ancestors became accomplished hunters. By then, hominids had evolved through *Homo habilis* and *Homo erectus*, had begun using stone tools, and had domesticated fire. This last was an important antecedent for meat eating, since cooking makes meat more palatable. The importance of dietary meat also increased at this time because the climate became cooler and drier in the preglacial era. During this period, "plant foods became more sparse," while "grazing animals on open grassy savannahs proliferated."[3] The development of language made hunting large animals easier, for it could be carried out cooperatively by groups of individuals as they communicated with one another.

Evidence for a hominid shift from being primarily herbivorous to being increasingly carnivorous comes from archeological research at prehistoric living sites. Animal bones have been found with "distinctive cut-marks and hammer indentations characteristic of butchering and marrow extraction," according to Tony McMichael's *Human Frontiers, Environments and Disease*:

> Anthropologists think that early humans probably came to rely on meat for around one-quarter of their daily calories. Meat intake not only provided energy; it supplied the full range of amino acids (the building blocks of proteins) and some important micronutrients (such as trace elements and vitamin B12) that were deficient in a vegetarian diet. In those precarious dietary circumstances, a modest meat intake would have significantly aided survival. It would also have consolidated cooperative hunting and food sharing. . . . The evidence, while still contentious, points increasingly to a Pleistocene in which early humans became serious hunters and big meat-eaters.[4]

By the late Paleolithic period, humans had become highly dependent on meat for sustenance. Recent study of bone chemistry of Neanderthals "overwhelmingly points to the Neanderthals behaving as top-level carnivores, obtaining almost all of their dietary protein from animal sources; . . . protein from plants was insignificant."[5] The importance of dietary protein at this time can also be measured by the size of humans. According to experts on Paleolithic nutrition, "*Homo sapiens sapiens*, who enjoyed an abundance of animal protein thirty thousand years ago, were an average of six inches taller than their descendants who lived after the development of farming," when meat consumption declined.[6]

Given this immense meat consumption, why didn't Paleolithic humans all succumb to heart attacks? One reason is that free-living animals have a much lower fat content in their muscles than do domesticated animals, and its composition is different; "wild game contains over five times more polyunsaturated fat per gram than is found in domestic livestock."[7] Thus, even though Paleolithic humans were eating large quantities of meat, it contained much less fat, and healthier forms of fat, than meat from domesticated animals.

In addition to hunting animals for meat, Paleolithic humans used animals for their skins and bones. Animal skins were early humans' primary source of protection from the cold. This became especially important during the four glacial periods between six hundred thousand and fifteen thousand years ago. At their peak, ice covered all of northern Europe as far south as central Germany and France, and the landscape was cold tundra, with little vegetation except during the summer months. The availability of skins of bison, aurochs (wild cattle), deer, ibex, wild sheep, bear, beaver, foxes, and other mammals largely determined whether humans survived or not. Humans also needed the bones of animals for making tools. Awls, harpoons, fish hooks, scrapers, and needles were fashioned from animal bones for at least seventy thousand years and were essential for hunting, fishing, butchering the catch, and sewing clothing.

In addition, at some point during the last hundred thousand years, *Homo sapiens* developed self-awareness. This may have been a consequence of the evolution of the frontal lobes of the brain or, as argued by Richard Klein in *The Dawn of Human Culture*, a genetic mutation.[8] From that time onward, animals became incorporated into humans' philosophic view of the world and their place within it. Animals thus began to play a major role in the creation myths of many cultures and continue even now to be incorporated into the ancestor stories and social structure of family and group organizations. An example of this is the role of animals in totems and clan identification among Native Americans along North America's northwest coast. One may argue that the use of animals as symbols for fraternal organizations, colleges, and sports teams is an extension of this group identity.

The late Paleolithic period, therefore, witnessed a major revolution in the relationship between humans and other animals. Following their divergence from chimpanzees, hominids had interacted minimally with other animals for five million years. Then, over a period of one million years, humans evolved increasingly as hunters, culminating in the late Paleolithic period, when hunting became the major human activity.

Thus emerged humans as hunters. For millions of years, hominids had merely watched other animals from afar. The new relationship required hunters to pursue and kill the animals. Knowledge of the animals' habits increased chances of success in the hunt, and for this reason it has been said that "the study of animal behavior is among the oldest of human endeavors."[9] Animals took on new meaning for Paleolithic humans. Bison and horses, viewed on the plains, became the Paleolithic equivalent of a McDonald's golden arch. A passing gazelle may have evoked the same reaction that a sign for Kentucky Fried Chicken does today.

The relationship between Paleolithic humans and animals is most clearly illustrated by the animal paintings, drawings, and etchings by Paleolithic artists in caves of southern France and northern Spain. In France's Chauvet cave, discovered in 1994, some of the paintings are thirty-two thousand years old. One panel shows four horses running side by side, another depicts ten lions moving toward some bison, and yet another has two rhinoceroses squared off to fight. France's Lascaux cave has a panel with five deer swimming across a river and, elsewhere, a remarkable deer with nine-point antlers, painted with red ocher from iron oxide. But Lascaux cave is best known for its Hall of the Bulls, a fifty-foot-long semicircular frieze painted seventeen thousand years ago. The animals are aurochs, the wild ancestors of contemporary cattle, and the artist needed scaffolding to paint them on the ceiling. One bull is sixteen feet long. Picasso, after visiting Lascaux, commented: "We have invented nothing!" [10]

In Spain's Altamira cave, the ceiling of the main hall, which has been called the Sistine Chapel of Paleolithic art, is one thousand square feet and covered with animals and geometric figures. Most prominent are "21 magnificently painted bison outlined and shaded in black, red bodies engraved in the glistening, creamy limestone. They crouch, lie down, shake their manes, charge across the ceiling, heads turned, tails flying, drilled eyes dark as coal." [11] The bison were engraved to emphasize eyes or other parts of their bodies. The artists took advantage of the natural rock contours of the ceiling so that one bison, whose head is turned to look back, appears three-dimensional because its head is painted on a rock outcropping. As described by one observer: "The figure develops in harmony in its surfaces; it leaps as if real and alive from the rugged surface of the rock. The fur, the beards, the manes of the bisons attain an almost tactile reality." [12]

Some of the bison appear so freshly painted and lifelike that in 1880, when Marcelino de Sautuola first published the results of his discovery of the cave, his claims that the paintings were Paleolithic in origin were derided. One skeptic, at an 1886 scientific meeting, claimed that "they are merely the expression of a mediocre follower of the Modern School," referring to emerging Impressionism. [13] It was not until 1902, after Sautuola had died, that the Altamira paintings were finally accepted as authentic.

This, then, was the new relationship between animals and humans. The Paleolithic cave paintings include no hills, no mountains, no natural scenery at all. Nor do they include any humans except for occasional stick figures in pursuit of the animals. The paintings represent Paleolithic humans' new and special relationship with animals — reverence, perhaps even worship. Sitting quietly in the main hall of Altamira cave, one is deeply impressed by the animals and by the people who painted them. It is an animal apotheosis. But with this new relationship came new diseases.

Taenia and Trichinosis

The animals Paleolithic humans killed, skinned, butchered, and ate were infected with an assortment of microbes, as all animals are. Since humans and the other animals had lived relatively separate lives for millions of years, humans had little previous exposure to most of these microbes. Their exposure now resulted in new infections, some harmless and some harmful, for Paleolithic humans. This can be illustrated by two macroparasite infestations, taenia and trichinosis, and five microbial diseases: anthrax, brucellosis, Q fever, tularemia, and glanders. All are examples of direct infection, as described in chapter 1, and all probably infected humans for the first time during the Paleolithic era. Such infections were part of the price humans began paying for their new relationship with animals. Humans hunted the animals, and the animals' microbes hunted the humans.

Recent studies have established that humans were first infected with *Taenia* tapeworms in Africa during the Paleolithic period. The source of the human infections was undercooked meat from wild cattle (aurochs) or wild boars.[14] *Taenia saginata* and *Taenia solium* infect humans when they ingest *Taenia* eggs in uncooked or undercooked beef or pork. In most cases, tapeworms cause no clinical symptoms, but in some individuals they cause abdominal pain, nausea and vomiting, and weight loss. A serious complication of *Taenia solium* is cysticercosis, in which numerous cysts go to the brain or eye, causing seizures or impaired vision. In developing countries, cysticercosis of the brain is the most common cause of acquired epilepsy, and even in Los Angeles, "neurocysticercosis was found in 10 percent of patients with seizures who went to an emergency room."[15]

Trichinosis is caused by *Trichinella spiralis*, a roundworm. Humans become infected when they eat uncooked or undercooked meat that contains cysts containing worm larva. Most humans have no symptoms unless they ingest a very large number of cysts; in such cases the cysts can infect the person's heart muscle or brain, and deaths from trichinosis have been reported. Wild boars, horses, and bears are all infected with *Trichinella spiralis* and could have been a source of infection for Paleolithic hunters.

Numerous other macroparasites are known, but most are of little or no clinical significance for humans. It seems likely that Paleolithic hunters would have encountered most of them as they skinned, butchered, and ate the animals of the African plains. Studies of the fossilized human excrement (coprolites) of early hunters have often found evidence of macroparasites.[16]

Anthrax, Brucellosis, and Q Fever

Anthrax, brucellosis, and Q fever are microbial diseases that were originally transmitted to early humans from wild ruminants, specifically the ancestors of cattle, sheep, and goats. These microbes have thus infected humans for thousands of years; in recent years, they have become prominent as possible agents for bioterrorism.

The Egyptians, Greeks, and Romans knew anthrax well. It achieved a unique place in history in 1877, when Robert Koch described it as the first microbe to be specifically linked to a disease. Anthrax spores live in the soil, where they are ingested by cattle and other grass-eating animals. The infected animals die, and their meat, hides, hair, and even bones can then spread the spores to humans.

The most common clinical form of human anthrax disease is the cutaneous form that produces black skin ulcers; untreated, it causes death in 25 percent of cases. Less common but much more serious is the systemic form in which anthrax spores are inhaled, producing initial flulike symptoms and almost always progressing to death within in a few days. Anthrax continues to occur among farm animals in many parts of the world, including the United States. An outbreak among cattle in North Dakota in 2000, for example, resulted in 157 animal deaths.[17]

Brucellosis is also an ancient disease; Hippocrates described it as Mediterranean fever. It continues to be widespread in the Mediterranean area even today; worldwide, approximately one-half million cases are reported each year, although it is rare in the United States. It is transmitted to humans from infected cattle or goats through butchering or by ingesting infected meat or unpasteurized milk, cream, or cheese. In animals it is an important cause of abortions, and in humans it is manifested by a relapsing fever (brucellosis is also called undulant fever), weakness, and muscle and joint pain. Untreated, it causes death in approximately 5 percent of cases.

Q fever acquired its name as an abbreviation for query fever by an Australian researcher investigating an outbreak of fever among slaughterhouse workers. Like anthrax and brucellosis, it is spread from cattle, sheep, and goats to humans and does not spread from person to person. It is caused by a rickett-sial type of bacteria and causes no symptoms in animals but may cause high fevers, pneumonia, hepatitis, or infection of the heart muscle in humans.

Tularemia and Glanders

Tularemia and glanders are also microbial diseases that were originally trans-mitted from animals to humans during the Paleolithic period. Tularemia comes from rabbits and squirrels, while glanders comes from horses and mules.

The bacteria that causes tularemia is transmitted to humans most often during the butchering and eating of infected rabbits or squirrels. Less often it is acquired from ticks or flies that have previously bitten an infected animal. Clini-cally, tularemia causes ulcers, enlarged lymph nodes, and occasionally pneu-monia. The mortality rate in untreated cases is approximately 10 percent.

Glanders is caused by bacteria carried by horses and mules. It can be acquired by eating the meat of infected animals, by butchering them, or merely through close contact with them, as has occurred among stable work-ers. In both horses and humans, glanders can cause skin ulcers (called *farcy* in horses), abscesses in internal organs, and pneumonia. Cases in humans have been described in which the person died less than three weeks after infection, "literally covered with pustules and ulcers."[18]

Glanders was known to the Greeks and remained an important disease until the gasoline engine replaced horses for transportation. For example, dur-ing the Civil War, Union and Confederate forces collected as many as 30,000 horses in large supply depots, and glanders spread quickly among them. At a Confederate depot in Lynchburg, Virginia, only 1,000 out of the 6,875 horses stabled there were said to be fit for service.[19] At a Union depot in Washington, D.C., 331 glanders-infected horses had to be shot in a single day.[20] The short-age of horses because of glanders created major problems for the armies on both sides. At the Battle of Chancellorsville in 1863, "more than one-fourth of the Confederate cavalry was without mounts."[21]

By the close of the Civil War, glanders had become widespread among horses on both the Union and Confederate sides. It had also presumably spread to many soldiers and was, along with typhoid, measles, tuberculosis, and other diseases, an additional source of mortality. When the Union and Confederate forces broke camp at the end of the war, they left behind many sick horses and mules "for the common people, both black and white. . . . Un-intentionally they opened a floodgate of disease upon the countryside." Other soldiers returned home accompanied by their sick animals in what has been called "a Civil War legacy."[22]

Paleolithic Microbes in the Modern Age

A recent synopsis of the biological and chemical agents most likely to be used for bioterrorism listed twelve microbes, including those that cause anthrax, brucellosis, Q fever, tularemia, and glanders[23]— legacies of animals hunted by Paleolithic peoples. It is interesting to speculate why some microbes that have infected humans for the longest time should be useful as agents of bioterrorism. All of them except brucellosis can be aerosolized and thereby spread through the air, all are hardy bacteria that can survive for long periods, and all are capable of causing disease in a wide variety of animals in addition to humans.

Anthrax is the best known and most feared among these. In October 2001, the United States became transfixed by anthrax when it was sent by mail to members of Congress and to a company in Florida. Inadvertently released from its envelope at a mail-sorting facility in Washington, D.C., anthrax killed two postal workers and caused illness in two dozen others. Anthrax is especially feared because its spores can be aerosolized, released into the air, and "if released in a fine-particle mist, . . . can ride air currents for 50 miles or more." A 1993 U.S. government assessment estimated that "if 220 pounds of aerosolized anthrax spores were released over Washington, D.C., between 130,000 and three million people would die."[24] Japanese troops are alleged to have used anthrax in this manner in China in the 1930s.

The microbe causing Q fever is also considered especially appropriate for bioterrorism because it spreads mainly by being blown through the air. For example, an outbreak in Switzerland infected 415 residents who lived along a road over which infected sheep were merely driven to pasture.[25] Thus, released into the air, Q fever could sicken thousands of people. Tularemia is of special interest to bioterrorists for the same reason — it also can be aerosolized and thereby spread by inhalation.

All five of these Paleolithic-era microbes have been, and presumably still are, under study by military researchers in the United States and elsewhere. All of them are also of interest to bioterrorists and have been used as agents of germ warfare.

The Germans used glanders, for example, in World War I to kill horses and mules destined for the Allied forces in Europe, where the animals were widely used for carrying supplies to the lines. Although technically still neutral, by 1915 the United States had become a principal source of war supplies for Britain and France, including thousands of horses and mules. The Germans evolved a plan to sabotage these equine supplies by infecting them with glanders before they were shipped abroad.

Brooklyn-born Anton "Tony" Dilger, the son of German immigrants, co-ordinated the plan. Trained in medicine at Johns Hopkins University in Baltimore, Dilger went to Germany before the war and was recruited as a German operative. In 1914 he returned to the United States and set up a laboratory in a house in Chevy Chase, Maryland, where he grew glanders bacteria in cultures.

To infect the horses and mules awaiting shipment to Europe, the Germans recruited Edward Felton, a stevedore in Baltimore. Dilger supplied glanders in small glass bottles that had "a piece of steel in the form of a needle with a sharp point . . . stuck in the underside of the cork, and the steel needle extended down in the liquid where the germs were." The Germans told Felton where to find the horses, and he recruited fellow stevedores to help him. According to testimony he later gave in court:

> I had about ten or twelve men working on these matters with me. We would work at it sometimes at night and sometimes in the daytime. A good many of the men were also doing other work and they made this extra money on the side. . . . We used rubber gloves and would put the germs in the horses by pulling out the stopper and jabbing the horses with the sharp point of the needle that had been down among the germs. We did a good bit of the work by walking along the fences that enclosed the horses and jabbing them when they would come up along the fence or lean over where we could get at them. We also spread the germs sometimes on their food and in the water they were drinking.[26]

Felton and his associates infected more than three thousand animals awaiting shipment to Europe, and these animals probably infected others. It was claimed that "several hundred military personnel were also affected."[27] The Germans regarded the sabotage efforts as so successful that "Dilger later went to St. Louis to establish a second lab there for the inoculation of Europe-bound horses and mules raised in Western states."[28] Germany may have extended its glanders program to Spain, Argentina, and other countries that were also supplying horses and mules to the Allied forces.[29]

The entry of the United States into the war in 1917 put an end to these German sabotage efforts. Dilger moved to Mexico, where, under an alias, he was said to be "the overseer of all German intelligence in Mexico."[30] Dilger later moved to Spain, where he died suddenly during the final months of the war. "It was whispered that he knew too much. It was a deadly poison that removed him — at least so it was intimated by a former German agent."[31]

The use of glanders in germ warfare was probably tested in extensive biowarfare research carried out by the Japanese in the 1930s and possibly in Soviet research during the Cold War. There are also allegations that Soviet forces used glanders to infect horses of resistance forces in Afghanistan during the 1982–1984 war.[32] In the United States, glanders has continued to be a subject of military research. Between November 1944 and September 1945, six cases of human glanders occurred among thirteen researchers working on the microbe at the army research facility at Fort Dietrich, Maryland.[33] In March 2000, a researcher at that facility developed severe glanders and had to be placed on a respirator before he was properly diagnosed and treated.[34] Thus, these ancient animal microbes that first infected Paleolithic hunters remain relevant today, primarily as agents of human destruction.

4

C H A P T E R

Humans as Farmers

Microbes Move into the Home

Directly or indirectly, every creature survives at some expense to others.
It stays alive only if it creates proteins; to do so, it must take in proteins
or the amino acids from which proteins are built. The ways one creature
makes another's protein its own range from predation to parasitism, but
all are paths to the same end.

ARNO KARLEN, *Man and Microbes*

NOBODY fully understands why humans domesticated crops and farm animals when they did. Changes in climate are only part of the explanation. Perhaps the continuing evolution of the human brain also played a role, allowing people to plan ahead and work together in ways that had not previously been possible. Whatever the reasons, the Neolithic revolution, as it is commonly called, changed the relationship between humans and other animals more profoundly than any other event in history.

By the beginning of the Neolithic period, hominids had spread broadly across the earth. They migrated from Africa into the Middle East and Asia approximately 1.7 million years ago and into Europe by 1 million years ago.[1] *Homo sapiens*, the only species of *Homo* that survived and that from which modern humans descend, spread widely around the earth beginning approximately one hundred thousand years ago and by the Neolithic period had reached Australia and South America. Whereas the total hominid population of eastern Africa had probably been no more than fifty thousand individuals before they began dispersing, by the Neolithic period the widely scattered humans numbered approximately five million.[2]

The climate in many areas of the earth became more hospitable to agriculture as the glaciers started to recede approximately fifteen thousand years ago. As the earth slowly warmed, grasslands and forests increasingly replaced the tundra across much of Europe, the Middle East, and Asia. One area especially rich in agricultural potential was the Fertile Crescent, which stretches for almost one thousand miles from what are now Israel and Palestine through Lebanon, Jordan, Syria, and southeastern Turkey into Iraq and Iran.

Growing wild in the Neolithic grasslands of the Fertile Crescent were ancestor grasses of wheat, barley, rye, lentils, and chick-peas.[3] According to Steve Olson in *Mapping Human History*: "Of the fifty-six grasses with the largest seeds, thirty-two grow in the Middle East, including wheat and barley. No other part of the world has more than a few such plants."[4] The upper reaches of the Tigris and Euphrates rivers, which cover part of northern Iraq and southeastern Turkey, were especially rich in the Neolithic founder crops and have been called "the cradle of agriculture."[5] There is evidence that agriculture developed independently in other areas of the world as well, including Southeast Asia, northern China, Africa, Papua New Guinea, Mexico, and Peru. The Fertile Crescent, however, was unique in having a wide variety of cultivatable plants, as well as wild olives, figs, grapes, dates, and apples.[6]

Agriculture, of course, did not develop at a single site or at a single time. Over hundreds, perhaps thousands, of years, humans picked the wild plants, harvested the edible parts, and discarded the seeds nearby. Inevitably some of the seeds grew into new plants. The cereal grains were ground, baked, and mixed with water to make an edible gruel. When gruel is allowed to stand, it uses bacteria to ferment and change into a type of beer. This development almost certainly added both impetus and enthusiasm to the agricultural revolution.

Neolithic people valued most the foods that they could store and that were good sources of calories — cereals such as wheat, barley, millet, rye, corn, and rice, as well as tubers such as potatoes, yams, and manioc (cassava).[7] Once a plant became well established as a source of food among one group of Neolithic farmers, its use spread to other parts of the world.

The use of increasingly sophisticated tools also encouraged the development and spread of agriculture during the Neolithic period. Recent experiments using a flint-bladed sickle demonstrate that one person could gather enough wild wheat in one hour to produce a kilo of grain. Experiments with a polished stone axe head report that "three men managed to clear 600 square yards of silver birch forest in 4 hours. . . . More than 100 trees were felled with one axe-head, which had not been sharpened for about 4,000 years."[8] Thus, Neolithic farmers were able to clear forested areas to enlarge the size of their gardens.

Domestication of Animals

At the same time that Neolithic people were domesticating plants, they were domesticating animals. The sequence of these two developments has been debated, but they probably occurred simultaneously and influenced each other. Using an animal to pull a plow, for example, doubled the area that could be cultivated by human power alone.[9] Similarly, the parts of cultivated crops that could not be used by humans could be fed to domesticated goats, pigs, and cattle.

For animals to become domesticated, according to Francis Galton, they must possess six characteristics: They must be "hardy" and able to adapt; they must be social; they must be "comfort-loving" and appreciate what humans have to offer them; they must be "useful" to those domesticating them; they must breed easily; and "they should be easy to tend." Only one animal does not follow these rules: "With the exception of the domestic cat, all domestic mammals are derived from wild species that are social rather than solitary in their behavior."[10]

The first animal *Homo sapiens* domesticated was the dog, approximately fourteen thousand years ago. Domestication may have occurred first in China or Japan, although once domesticated, dogs spread quickly throughout the settled world.[11] The process of domestication has been widely debated: Did humans domesticate wolves, or did wolves domesticate themselves?

Proponents of the first position argue that taming wolf pups is comparatively easy. In this scenario, early humans kept and bred those pups that were especially placid and submissive and then learned to use the tamed wolves to help hunt deer and other mammals and to warn of approaching enemies at night. The experiments of Soviet biologist D. K. Belyaev support this scenario. Belyaev, working with silver foxes, selected for breeding those foxes that showed the most "consistently tame behavior toward humans." Twenty years after the selective breeding began, "the results were astonishing." Belyaev's "tame-selected foxes were not just tame; they acted for all the world like domestic dogs. They approached familiar persons and licked their hands and faces. They barked like dogs. They even sought the attention of strangers by whining and wagging their tails. Their annual molting cycle was disrupted, and the females began to come into heat twice a year, like dogs, and unlike both foxes and wolves."[12]

Proponents of the alternate theory call attention to the evolution of both early humans and wolves "as social hunters" and point out that "during the glacial phases of the Upper Pleistocene, they had the same ubiquitous distribution and they preyed on the same herds of large mammals."[13] According to this scenario, wolves began hanging around human campsites to scavenge garbage and gradually became less fearful. These wolves were not being selected by humans but rather were selecting themselves: "These were animals that chose to hang around humans, and in so doing to isolate themselves from their wild counterparts by their own volition."[14] Over time, being social and hierarchical in nature, the wolves would have accepted the human social order as their own in exchange for food. As Stephen Budiansky summarized this scenario in *The Covenant of the Wild:* "In an evolutionary sense, domesticated animals chose us as much as we chose them."[15] Rudyard Kipling portrayed such a scene in his 1912 *Just So Stories,* in which he has a woman throw a "roasted mutton-bone" to "Wild Thing out of the Wild Woods":

> Wild Dog gnawed the bone, and it was more delicious than anything he had ever tasted, and he said, "O my Enemy and Wife of my Enemy, give me another."
> The Woman said, "Wild Thing out of the Wild Woods, help my Man to hunt through the day and guard this Cave at night, and I will give you as many roast bones as you need."[16]

Sheep and goats were the next animals to become domesticated. The wild ancestors of both lived in the Fertile Crescent, especially in the Zagros Mountains in what is now western Iraq. Domestication would not have been difficult, since both sheep and goats follow a dominant leader. They also have relatively placid natures, breed easily in captivity, and eat a wide variety of shrubs and grasses. Evidence that suggests the domestication of sheep has been found at a site in northern Iraq that dates to almost eleven thousand years ago. Goat domestication in this area apparently began about ten thousand years ago.[17] The problem with fixing such dates with any certainty is one of definitions. Does the simple herding of wild goats or sheep qualify as domestication? Or confining them to fenced areas? Breeding them while in captivity, or breeding selectively so as to enhance certain characteristics?

Goats were an especially valuable commodity in the ancient world and continue to be so today in many parts of the developing world. As Juliet Clutton-Brock notes: "The goat can provide both the primitive peasant farmer and the nomadic pastoralist with all his physical needs, clothing, meat, and milk as well as bone and sinew for artifacts, tallow for lighting, and dung for fuel and manure."[18] In addition, goat's milk can be made into cheese, its wool used for clothing, and its skins used for both clothing and water containers. It is thus not surprising that the five-thousand-year-old man discovered in 1991 in a glacier in the Alps was wearing a jacket and leggings made of goat- and deerskins. Goats may have also been helpful to Neolithic farmers in clearing land for planting by eating shrubs and low-hanging trees. Since goats eat plants that sheep and cows will not, they are very hardy and adaptable and can be raised in a wider variety of environments, including those that are semi-desert.

Humans next domesticated pigs and cattle. Their ancestors, wild boars and aurochs, were widely distributed across the Middle East, Asia, and Europe, so domestication could theoretically have occurred in many places over a broad geographic area. DNA analyses from contemporary animals, however, suggest that for both pigs and cattle, "modern livestock derived from a small number of animals domesticated in just a few places 8,000 to 10,000 years ago."[19]

Domesticated pigs are relatively easy to maintain. They eat almost anything, produce two litters a year, and provide a steady supply of protein as ham, pork, and bacon. Although ancient Semitic peoples and modern-day followers of Jewish and Islamic rituals shun pigs as unclean for food, they are highly valued in many Asian and Pacific Island cultures. In some parts of Papua New Guinea, for example, pigs are the major means for counting one's wealth, and it is not uncommon for a woman to suckle a piglet at her breast alongside her own child.

In contrast, the circumstances that led early humans to domesticate wild aurochs as cattle are difficult to imagine, for the animals were not only six feet high but "fierce, swift and agile."[20] They would certainly have been more difficult than pigs or goats to herd from village to village and, if left to roam freely, would have trampled the grain in the gardens and fields.

Nevertheless, Neolithic humans discovered the immense value of domesticated aurochs. Cattle can provide meat, milk, butter, and cheese as food. Their horns are useful as weapons and their dried hides make good shields, both valuable in warfare. The hides can also be used for making shoes and clothing. Cattle dung can be burned as fuel, used as fertilizer, and used in pastes for the building of huts, and cattle fat can be burned as tallow. Cattle may also be used to thrash grain by walking on it, pull carts, and turn wheels to bring water from wells. Frederick Zeuner, in *A History of Domesticated Animals*, claimed that, after dogs, "the domestication of cattle was the most important step ever taken by man in the direction of exploitation of the animal world."[21] Given these contributions, it is not surprising that many societies have revered, even worshipped, cattle.

Horses were domesticated next, approximately five thousand years ago, in Turkestan, Ukraine, and southern Russia, where wild horses were abundant.[22] In contrast to pigs and cattle, DNA analyses of modern horses suggest that they were domesticated at multiple places and at different times.[23] Horses were probably originally domesticated as an additional source of meat, but their value as transportation soon became apparent.

The successful domestication of goats, sheep, pigs, cattle, and horses—

referred to as the "Big Five"[24]—was an enormous advantage for Neolithic people, providing them with a reliable supply of food, clothing, and transportation. Selective breeding rapidly produced groups of animals with special characteristics, and "both the Babylonian and the Ancient Egyptian civilizations had developed definitive breeds of dogs, cattle, and sheep by the beginning of the second millennium B.C."[25]

The idea of domesticating animals spread quickly across the world and in some cases was accomplished independently. Oxen, yaks, water buffalo, gaur, banteng, reindeer, camels, donkeys, elephants, and alpacas were domesticated for tasks such as carrying loads; pulling plows, wagons, or sleds; or turning wheels to pump water from wells. Ducks, geese, and turkeys were domesticated for food; cats, as we will see later, were domesticated by Egyptians to keep rodents away from the grain or simply as pets. The Egyptians, in fact, were so enthusiastic about domesticating animals that they also tried, though unsuccessfully, to domesticate antelopes, gazelles, hyenas, and monkeys.[26]

Enter the Microbes

Peoples of the Neolithic period, then, profoundly and permanently altered the relationship between animals and humans. Animals that early hominids had watched from afar for millions of years, and Paleolithic humans had hunted for thousands of years, now grazed peacefully in the backyard. In the past, animals and humans had essentially been equals; after domestication, that was no longer true. As James Serpell observed in *In the Company of Animals:* "This essentially egalitarian relationship disappeared with the advent of domestication. The domestic animal is dependent for survival on its human owner. The human becomes the overlord and master, the animals his servants and slaves."[27] This new relationship between animals and humans was symbolized by how humans depicted animals. As one art historian observed: "The altered relationship to the animal world of man as hunter and man as farmer was inevitable and seems to account for differences between the commanding bulls and bison of Lascaux . . . and the tiny, toy-like horned animals found on Neolithic sites such as Hăbăşeşti, or the heads attached to Neolithic and Bronze Age pots" several centuries later.[28]

A consequence of the domestication of animals was a marked increase in intimacy between animals and humans. Sheep, goats, pigs, and cows were often housed immediately adjacent to, or under the same roof as, Neolithic farmers. In agrarian areas of the developing world, it is still not unusual to find several animals sharing one-room living quarters with an extended human family. Even in Western nations, the separation of living quarters for farm animals and humans is a relatively recent phenomenon.

Following domestication, therefore, animals not only entered the home but also became part of the family. According to Keith Thomas: "Sheep or pigs were not usually given individual names, but cows always were, . . . like Marigold or Lily." Furthermore, "shepherds know the faces of their sheep as well as those of their neighbors."[29] Such animals were usually the family's most valuable possessions, as well as its main sources of milk and meat. The animals were nursed when they were sick and midwifed, as needed, when giving birth. The extent of the intimacy between domesticated animals and humans is also symbolized by humans' drinking of the milk of goats and cows. As Joanna Swabe has pointed out: "The practice of drinking cow's milk, particularly by human babies, . . . created an intense bond between humans and other animals; by seeking the milk of another species to nourish their young, humans were effectively using cattle as wet-nurses."[30]

The new relationship between animals and humans led to many new human diseases. The animals Neolithic people domesticated were carrying a variety of bacteria, viruses, and protozoa that had evolved with the animals over thousands, even millions, of years. Putting the previously wild animals into pens and other enclosures facilitated the dissemination of microbes within each species. Placing different animal species, such as sheep and goats, within the same enclosures encouraged the spread of microbes across species, sometimes producing new and different strains of the microbes.

Many of the microbes inevitably spread from the domesticated animals to humans. They spread when Neolithic people ingested the meat or milk products of the animals. They spread through the air when animals were housed within human dwellings. They spread through animal feces, which were deposited close to human dwellings, used as building material, burned as fuel, and spread as fertilizer on Neolithic farmers' crops, and which contaminated water supplies being used by humans. The microbes spread when dogs or other domesticated animals licked or bit people. They spread by being carried by flies, ticks, mosquitoes, fleas, or other vectors from the domesticated animals to humans living close by. And they spread when humans had sexual contact with animals, as has occasionally occurred throughout history and is depicted in prehistoric art.[31] Indeed, in the years following the initial domestication of animals, humans were heavily exposed to a multitude of animal microbes to which they had previously been exposed only minimally or not at all.

Ulcers, Whooping Cough, and Smallpox

We are still learning the microbial consequences of the domestication of animals, and as the genomes of additional microbes are characterized by nucleotide sequencing in coming years, we will gain a more complete picture. What is already clear is that many important human diseases can be traced to bacteria, viruses, and protozoa that were first transmitted from animals to humans during the Neolithic revolution.

Peptic ulcers in humans are an example. They are caused by an erosion of the lining of the stomach or the duodenum, the first segment of the small intestine. The main symptoms are abdominal pain, usually sharply localized to the midabdomen. Untreated, ulcers are a common cause of gastrointestinal bleeding, which makes people vomit blood or pass blood in their feces. Ulcers, especially of the duodenal variety, can also perforate the wall of the intestine, thereby allowing infectious organisms into the abdominal cavity, causing generalized infection (peritonitis). Bleeding or perforated ulcers may cause death.

Throughout most of the twentieth century, the causes of peptic ulcers were widely believed to be "hurry, worry and curry."[32] Psychotherapy was commonly recommended for patients with ulcers as a means of reducing stress. In 1982, however, Australian researchers proved that most peptic ulcers are caused by a spiral-shaped bacteria, *Helicobacter pylori*, which had long been known to be present in human stomachs but whose significance had not been appreciated.[33] This discovery has profoundly changed our understanding of peptic ulcers.

Approximately 50 percent of the world's population is infected with *Helicobacter pylori*, making it "one of the most common bacterial infections in humans."[34] It spreads from person to person in childhood, more quickly in crowded households.[35] The bacteria may possibly also be spread by contaminated water or by flies. We are not certain why it causes peptic ulcers in some individuals and not in others, but genetic predisposition, as described in chapter 1, certainly plays some role.

The origins of *Helicobacter pylori* are still under debate. Some observers have suggested that it is an heirloom infection and has infected hominids for millions of years, while others suggest that it was transmitted from animals to humans in the more recent past. Many animals carry spiral-shaped bacteria that are closely related to *Helicobacter pylori*. Dogs, cats, horses, cows, pigs, sheep, and some primates are thought to carry *Helicobacter pylori* itself.[36] Suggestions that it spreads from animals to humans have come from studies of abattoir workers and employees of meat-processing plants, who have an unusually high incidence of infection.[37]

The leading animal candidate as the origin of human *Helicobacter pylori* is the sheep. In rural Sardinia, it has been reported that 98 percent of shepherds are infected with this bacteria, an infection rate more than twice that of Sardinians who are not shepherds.[38] *Helicobacter pylori* is also commonly present in sheep's milk, which shepherds often drink raw.[39] Studies in Sardinia have shown that children in rural areas who are exposed to dogs, many of which are used to herd sheep, have a higher rate of *Helicobacter pylori* infection than children not exposed to dogs.[40] Additional support for the association of *Helicobacter pylori* with sheep comes from studies of shepherds in Poland and from studies in South America that show that children exposed to sheep have a higher rate of infection.[41]

The emerging hypothesis regarding the origin of *Helicobacter pylori*, then, is that "sheep were the ancestral host of the bacteria and that it entered the human population after domestication of sheep."[42] Sheep have been very closely tied to humans since domestication, as illustrated by the widespread imagery of sheep and shepherds in the Bible.

Another example of a human disease that was probably originally transmitted from animals to humans after animals were domesticated is whooping cough, or pertussis. Before public health measures improved and use of a vaccine became widespread in the first half of the twentieth century, whooping cough was one of the most feared childhood diseases. Even today it results in approximately thirty-five thousand deaths per year worldwide, most of them in infants.

The bacteria that causes human whooping cough, *Bordetella pertussis*, is very closely related to a bacteria (*Bordetella parapertussis*) that occurs in both humans and sheep, and also to a bacteria (*Bordetella bronchiseptica*) that occurs in pigs, dogs, cats, rabbits, rats, horses, and some primates, occasionally including humans. For many years, it was assumed that *Bordetella pertussis* came originally from the sheep bacteria, but recent studies have shown that this is not the case.[43] Instead it now seems likely that human whooping cough came from pigs.[44]

Pigs are reservoirs for many human diseases in addition to whooping cough. For example, the nipah virus is carried by pigs and also affects dogs, cats, horses, and bats. In 1998–1999, an outbreak of encephalitis in Malaysia killed 105 of the 265 people infected with this virus, most of whom had come in close contact with pigs. The outbreak was brought under control by killing one million pigs, but smaller outbreaks have since occurred in Singapore and Bangladesh. Pigs also play a crucial role in the evolution of new strains of the influenza virus (see chapter 9).

One of the most important diseases that appears to have been transmitted to humans following the domestication of animals is smallpox. Intimately associated with the history of the New World, smallpox first devastated the Aztecs and Incas in Mexico and Peru, then wiped out entire tribes of North American Indians. Smallpox also figures prominently as a potential microbe for bioterrorism and was one of the first microbes so used; in 1763 British officer Lord Jeffrey Amherst ordered his troops to give smallpox-infected blankets to Native Americans to deliberately infect them.[45]

The origins of smallpox have long been debated. The virus that causes it is a member of the orthopoxvirus family. This family includes the monkey-pox virus, which affects many rodents and which recently infected pet prairie dogs in an outbreak in the United States (see chapter 7). Recent research, however, suggests that the smallpox virus did not come from the monkeypox virus.[46] The orthopoxvirus family also includes the cowpox virus, which not only affects cows but also is especially common in members of the cat family and may cause mild infections in humans.[47] A third closely related virus is the buffalopox virus, which infects water buffalo, cattle, and occasionally humans.[48] Water buffalo were first domesticated in Southeast Asia,[49] and it is perhaps significant that, approximately three thousand years ago, the earliest recorded cases of smallpox also appeared in this region.[50] Ongoing molecular research should soon provide a definitive answer regarding the animal origins of the smallpox virus.

Regardless of the origin of human smallpox, it was the relatedness of the smallpox virus to another member of the orthopoxvirus family, the vaccinia virus, that allowed the development of immunizations that have essentially eliminated naturally occurring cases of smallpox from the face of the earth. The recent fears concerning the spread of smallpox by means of bioterrorism have highlighted the importance of vaccinia in terms of providing protection to the general population.

Tuberculosis

Of all microbes bequeathed to humans as a consequence of animal domestication, the deadliest was the bacterium that causes tuberculosis. Currently, tuberculosis kills nearly two million people each year worldwide, and it has "probably killed 100 million people over the past 100 years."[51] It was for good reason that John Bunyan, in 1680, called tuberculosis "the captain of all these men of death."[52]

Even though almost all cases of human tuberculosis are now spread from person to person, humans were probably first infected by contact with domesticated animals. Robert Koch in 1882 identified the tuberculosis bacterium that infects humans as *Mycobacterium tuberculosis*. A closely related member of the same family is *Mycobacterium bovis*, which causes an important disease of cattle and which can also infect sheep, goats, pigs, rabbits, cats, and other animals. Molecular studies have shown that these two bacteria are almost identical.[53]

For many years it was believed that *Mycobacterium tuberculosis*, the cause of human disease, had evolved from *Mycobacterium bovis* when cattle were domesticated. Recent studies, however, suggest a more complex story: Both bacteria evolved from a common ancestor.[54] The studies have also shown that the *Mycobacterium bovis* strains that infect cattle and goats differ from each other—the goat strain has a molecular structure more closely related to human *Mycobacterium tuberculosis* than has the cattle strain.[55] The authors of one study concluded: "Considering the results shown here, it is tempting to speculate that the immediate missing-link ancestor of *Mycobacterium tuberculosis* . . . may be the goat *M. bovis* strains and not the cattle *M. bovis* strains, as was proposed previously."[56] This hypothesis would also be consistent with the fact that goats can become infected with human *Mycobacterium tuberculosis* but cattle cannot.[57]

The ancestors of both *Mycobacterium tuberculosis* and *Mycobacterium bovis*, then, may have been bacteria carried by wild bezoar goats in the Fertile Crescent. The bacteria would have evolved into the human strain as humans domesticated goats, sharing living quarters with them, eating their meat, and drinking their milk.

The sharing of living quarters between humans and animals was an especially important facet of the evolution of human tuberculosis. *Mycobacteria* are unusual microbes insofar as they do not usually cause disease except when humans or other animals are crowded together. This has been clearly demonstrated in cattle: "It is a universal experience that the incidence of bovine tuberculosis increases in proportion to the density of the cattle population, i.e., to the size of the herds and the space allotted to the cattle when they are kept indoors."[58] This phenomenon has also been observed in American buffalo; when roaming unconfined in a large national park, they were found to be virtually free of bovine tuberculosis, whereas buffalo confined and mixed with cattle were reported to be heavily infected.[59] Similarly, monkeys that live in the wild are free of tuberculosis, whereas "the monkey in captivity is the most susceptible of all animals to tuberculosis."[60] The events that led to the evolution of human tuberculosis, then, were not only the domestication of goats and other animals, but also the crowding together of the animals and humans into the confined spaces of homes.

The King's Evil

The earliest claim for the origins of human tuberculosis has been from human remains in Germany approximately seven thousand years old. Definite tuberculosis was diagnosed in a mummified corpse in Egypt approximately three thousand years old; ancient Egypt may even have had a large sanitarium for treating the disease.[61] Tuberculosis was also widespread in ancient Greece and Rome and spread in ancient times to North America, probably by way of the Bering land bridge; proof lies in the discovery of *Mycobacterium tuberculosis* in a Peruvian mummy dated to before the arrival of Columbus.[62]

One manifestation of tuberculosis is enlargement of lymph glands in the neck, commonly called *scrofula*. Beginning in the Middle Ages in France and England, it became widely believed that a king's touch could heal scrofula. People widely referred to scrofula as "the king's evil," and by the reign of Henry VII in the late fifteenth century, the ceremony of touching scrofulous individuals had become highly ritualized, with "prayers recited by priests, stroking of both sides of the face with both hands by the king, hanging a gold piece about the patient's neck, and closing prayers and a blessing."[63] In 1606, Shakespeare included a description of this ceremony in *Macbeth*:

> *Strangely visited people,*
> *All swoln and ulcerous, pitiful to the eye,*
> *The mere despair of surgery, he cures;*
> *Hanging a golden stamp about their necks,*
> *Put on with holy prayers.*
>
> (ACT 4, SCENE 3)

Easter Sunday, Pentecost, and the Feast of Michaelmas were especially favored times. Given the exposure of kings to scrofulous individuals, it is not surprising that Henry VII, his eldest son, Arthur, and his grandson, Edward VII, are all thought to have died from tuberculosis.[64] Their deaths played a major role in the history of England. The death of Arthur in 1502, before he could inherit the throne, resulted in the ascendancy of his brother, Henry VIII, who eventually led England out of the Catholic Church when the pope refused to grant him a divorce from his first wife, Catherine. The death of Edward VII in 1553 led to the ascendancy of his Catholic half-sister Mary, whose attempts to reinstitute the Catholic Church in England led to much civil strife and retribution, earning her the appellation "Bloody Mary." Religious strife continued in England until Mary's death and the ascendancy of her Protestant, and more tolerant, half-sister Elizabeth in 1558.

In the seventeenth century, tuberculosis appears to have markedly increased in incidence. By 1650, it was thought to account for 20 percent of deaths in England and Wales, with approximately one-quarter of the entire European population being infected.[65] Between 1662 and 1682, King Charles II is recorded to have touched ninety-two thousand individuals with scrofula. At a ceremony of touching in 1684, seven persons were trampled to death while attempting to reach the king.[66]

Seventeenth-century England presented ideal conditions for the spread of tuberculosis. In the previous century, the population of London had tripled, so crowding was endemic; many people lived several to a room. Recurring visitations of the plague, including the 1665 epidemic that killed one-quarter of London's population, weakened people's immune systems, so they had less resistance to infections. It was a chaotic century, both socially and politically, with civil war and an unstable monarchy.

Tuberculosis continued to ravage Europe during the eighteenth and nineteenth centuries as the industrial revolution brought additional urbanization and household crowding. In colder seasons, people crowded around the fire and kept windows tightly shut, thereby exposing everyone in the house to microbes carried by any one of them. Many houses had no windows to open. In 1696 in England, and later in France, the government instituted a tax on glass windows, which were still considered luxuries; many landlords simply bricked up the windows rather than pay the tax.[67]

The death rate from tuberculosis continued to climb, especially in cities and in crowded institutions. By 1780 in England, more than one person in every hundred died from tuberculosis each year.[68] In an English orphanage, 169 out of 172 children were diagnosed with scrofula; in Paris, tuberculosis was found to be the cause of death in more than one-third of all cases brought to autopsy.[69]

"Blood Was Its Avatar"

At about this time, tuberculosis began to be romanticized. Individuals afflicted with "consumption," as it was called, were thought to be endowed with "a peculiar quality of spirituality, even with creative genius."[70] This view prevailed especially among the literati of that period.

Poet John Keats was one of many writers and artists who became infected. When he was fourteen, Keats's mother died from tuberculosis after he had spent many weeks caring for her. At twenty-three, Keats nursed his brother, who was also dying from tuberculosis. Just over a year later, Keats coughed up blood for the first time; trained as a physician, he immediately knew its meaning. He said to a friend: "I know the color of that blood; — it is arterial blood; —I cannot be deceived in that color; that drop of blood is my death warrant. I must die." Percy Bysshe Shelley, who also had tuberculosis and was Keats's close friend, wrote to him: "This consumption is a disease particularly fond of people who write good verse as you have done."[71] Shortly thereafter Keats wrote *Ode to a Nightingale,* in which "youth grows pale, and specter-thin, and dies":

> *Darkling I listen; and for many a time*
> *I have been half in love with easeful Death.*[72]

One year later, Keats died at the age of twenty-five.

During the 1820s in Germany, Johann Wolfgang von Goethe was completing *Faust,* and in Scotland, Sir Walter Scott was publishing a new novel almost every year; both had suffered from tuberculosis. In 1827, young Frederic Chopin's sister developed fulminating tuberculosis and, eight years later, he too began showing the symptoms of the disease that eventually led to his death. In Paris during the 1840s, two young women who would become operatic heroines died from tuberculosis. One, Alphonsine Plessis, was a well-known courtesan who became the subject of an 1848 novel and eventually, as Violetta, the heroine of Giuseppe Verdi's 1853 opera *La Traviata*. The other young woman also became the subject of a novel, *Scene da "La Vie de Bohème,"* later adapted by Giacomo Puccini as *La Bohème*. At the end of the opera, a thin, pale, and consumptive Mimi asks Rudolfo, "Am I still beautiful?" He replies: "As beautiful as dawn."[73]

In England at this time, the closing scenes in the Brontë family tragedy were being played out. By the late 1840s, the two youngest children had died from tuberculosis at the family parsonage in Haworth, and the other four were to follow. Branwell died in 1848, followed by Emily, who had recently completed *Wuthering Heights*. A few months later Anne, who had published *Agnes Gray*, died in 1849. Charlotte, author of *Jane Eyre*, was the last to die, in 1855. One can visit their home today and see the table they sat around together as they wrote. From their front porch, the view of the Yorkshire hills must look as it did then; goats graze quietly on the hillside, unaware of the role their ancestors may have played in such human tragedies.

In the United States, where Edgar Allan Poe was publishing poems and short stories, his wife and foster mother had both died from tuberculosis, and Poe himself was infected. In "The Masque of the Red Death," Poe described tuberculosis as "a thief in the night. . . . Blood was its Avatar and seal." When the "Red Death" appears, the hour is sounded by "the brazen lungs of the clock," and after everyone has died, "the life of the ebony clock went out."[74] In New England at about this time, Ralph Waldo Emerson and Henry David Thoreau were sharing a house; both had tuberculosis, which Emerson survived but Thoreau did not.

In the late nineteenth century, Fyodor Dostoyevsky in Russia wrote about tuberculosis in *The House of the Dead*. Dostoyevsky's wife had died from the disease, as Dostoyevsky did later. Russian playwright Anton Chekhov suffered from tuberculosis for many years and eventually died from it. Like Chekhov, Robert Louis Stevenson suffered from tuberculosis for most of his life. He described the experience of having tuberculosis as being "like an enthusiast leading about with him a stolid, indifferent tourist."[75] At one point, Stevenson's doctors splinted his right arm to his chest to try to keep his tuberculous right lung quiescent; Stevenson then learned to write with his left hand. In 1880, Stevenson was hospitalized in Davos, Switzerland, at a tuberculosis sanitarium; there he wrote much of *Treasure Island*.[76]

Thirty years later, the wife of Thomas Mann was hospitalized at Davos for the treatment of her tuberculosis. While visiting his wife in 1912, Mann himself was diagnosed with the disease. He remained at Davos only long enough to make notes for his novel about a tuberculosis sanitarium, *The Magic Mountain.*

Late nineteenth-century tuberculosis affected artists as well as writers. Edvard Munch's mother died from tuberculosis when he was five, and his sister died from the disease when he was fourteen. He portrayed his despair in several paintings, including *The Dead Mother, Death in the Sickroom,* and, according to some critics, *The Scream.*

The scourge of tuberculosis continued to follow writers into the twentieth century. Franz Kafka, Katherine Mansfield, Thomas Wolfe, and George Orwell all died from it, the last shortly after completing *Nineteen Eighty-Four.* Terminally ill with the disease, D. H. Lawrence wrote in *The Ship of Death:* "Piecemeal the body dies, and the timid soul / has her footing washed away, as the dark flood rises."[77]

In the latter half of the twentieth century, following the discovery of streptomycin and other antituberculosis drugs, there was hope of controlling, perhaps even eradicating, this ancient scourge. In the 1980s, increasingly widespread drug-resistant strains of the bacteria, along with the AIDS epidemic, extinguished this hope. As the immune system of AIDS patients loses its ability to fight infections, *Mycobacterium tuberculosis* is a major invader; thus, 38 percent of new cases of tuberculosis in sub-Saharan Africa now occur in individuals with AIDS.[78]

Tuberculosis remains a major threat in the United States as well. In Minnesota in 1992, a man with untreated tuberculosis infected forty-one patrons and employees of a bar he frequented.[79] In Maryland in 1993, a university student with untreated tuberculosis infected thirty-three friends and acquaintances; investigators concluded that she had been "more infectious than the average child with measles."[80] Tuberculosis has become an especially prominent problem among individuals who are homeless and living in public shelters; in Seattle in 2002, thirty such cases were diagnosed.[81]

5

CHAPTER

Humans as Villagers

Microbes in the Promised Land

> *Nor is it a new thing for man to invent an existence that he imagines to be*
> *above the rest of life; this has been his most consistent intellectual exertion*
> *down the millennia. As illusion, it has never worked out to his satisfaction*
> *in the past, any more than it does today. Man is embedded in nature.*
>
> LEWIS THOMAS, *The Lives of a Cell*

PALEOLITHIC hunters were remarkably isolated. For hundreds of thousands of years, they lived in small, extended family bands, often moving seasonally to follow the migrations of animals they hunted. According to Karlen's *Man and Microbes*, the hunters "lived in bands of probably a few dozen, perhaps a hundred at most, . . . seldom exceeding a density of one person per square mile."[1] Because of their sparse distribution, contact between groups was infrequent. During an entire lifetime, an individual would probably have interacted with no more than a few hundred other individuals.

Neolithic farmers at first were also widely scattered. However, as the domestication of grains and animals progressed, a reliable supply of food was increasingly available in a single location. Individual families began settling closer to each other in hamlets and small villages, often living in homes clustered together and farming the surrounding fields. Such villages afforded mutual protection against wild animals, which would have been attracted to the domesticated animals. The villages also offered some protection against other human groups that might try to steal their grain or animals. Most villages consisted of three hundred people or less. During an entire lifetime, an individual would probably have interacted at most with only a few thousand others.

Over time, some of the villages grew to become towns. By nine thousand years ago, Zawi Chemi Shanidar in northern Iraq, Jericho in Israel, and Catalhöyük in Turkey had all achieved town status. Jericho, for example, had a population of approximately two thousand people and had a wall around it for protection. In Catalhöyük, the homes were substantial: "The living rooms had built-in furniture consisting of benches and platforms, as well as hearths and ovens, all made from earth and plaster. Groups of rooms, each with a storeroom, were centered around shrines."[2]

A relatively stable food supply and settled population made it easier to raise children, and so beginning approximately ten thousand years ago, humans began proliferating more quickly. It has been estimated that the world's population was no greater than five million when domestication of grains and animals began. Within four thousand years, the world's population had increased tenfold, to approximately fifty million.[3] Towns grew accordingly, and a few merged with other nearby towns to create the first urban centers of eighty to one hundred thousand people. During an entire lifetime, an individual living in such an urban area may have interacted with as many as ten thousand others.

The urbanization of Neolithic people occurred first in Mesopotamia, which was watered by the Tigris and Euphrates rivers. Uruk, Ur, Lagash, Kish, and Erech were significant centers of population; Erech's walls encompassed two square miles.[4] In Egypt, urban centers such as Memphis and Thebes developed in the Nile Valley; in what is now Pakistan, along the Indus River, Mohenjo-Daro and Harappa became important centers of population. By approximately 4,500 years ago, each of these three river valleys "probably contained about three-quarters of a million people."[5]

A Microbial Feast

From the viewpoint of bacteria, viruses, and protozoa, village life offered many advantages. Closed and dark houses kept out sunlight, a powerful enemy of microbes. The houses also promoted the recirculation of stale air, so that microbes could move freely among human respiratory tracts, especially in crowded rooms. Permanent houses also promoted the accumulation of trash, garbage, and feces, which attracted mice, rats, mosquitoes, and flies, some of which moved permanently into the human dwellings. As Karlen described conditions: "The gardens of Babylon and temples of Egypt were emblems of urban glory, but the alleys in their shadows were choked with garbage. Homes reeked with fetid air and smoke. Vast amounts of human and animal wastes accumulated; water was drawn from contaminated wells, food harvested from tainted fields. Dirt and refuse drew every germ-bearing scavenger that flew, crept, or crawled."[6] Mosquitoes, flies, and other vectors fed on both humans and domesticated animals nearby. For microbes, which for millions of years had chased nomadic animals and hominids across open spaces, it was like sitting at a banquet table.

Predictably, the bringing of people together into villages, towns, and urban areas resulted in increasing microbial-caused infections. Studies of early settlements, for example, reveal that "the percentage of individuals displaying signs of infection doubled in the transition from hunting and gathering to intensive maize cultivation; . . . rates of infection were positively correlated with the size and permanence of the communities."[7]

The main reason increasing microbial infections follow an increasing density of people is that many microbes cannot exist without a minimum density of people or other animals. For example, "a strain of ear-nose-throat bacteria that persists for an average of four months may be sustained by a group of only 70 persons, while one that persists for only one month may require up to 500 persons if continuing transmission is to be achieved."[8] A sufficient population density is especially necessary for microbes that induce permanent immunity following initial infection. In such cases, there must be enough susceptible individuals who have never been infected to keep the microbe circulating; once it infects everyone, it simply dies out.

For such reasons, many infectious diseases increased in incidence as humans moved closer together in ever-increasing groups. Tuberculosis and smallpox are well-known examples, and evidence of both has been found in mummies from ancient Egypt. Less known are microbes that began to infect humans only when a sufficient number of people lived together.

Examples of this that everyone has experienced are human rhinoviruses, the most frequent causes of common colds. For many years, it was assumed that rhinoviruses had been originally transmitted to humans from horses, but more recently it has been shown that human rhinoviruses originated from bovine counterparts in cattle.[9] After transmission to humans, the rhinoviruses underwent mutations and specifically adapted to humans, as discussed in chapter 1. Thus, human rhinoviruses are no longer thought to be transmitted to humans from cattle but rather to circulate only among humans. To do this, they need a large group of people to act as a reservoir for the viruses and to keep the viruses from dying out. Such conditions exist only in towns and urban areas. Thus, human colds are a product of humans' both having domesticated cattle and then moving into villages and towns.

Measles

The best example of a microbe that requires a large number of people to survive is the measles virus, which was also originally transmitted to humans from cattle. Like human rhinoviruses, the measles virus no longer spreads from animals to humans but is instead transmitted exclusively from humans to humans. Since it confers permanent immunity following an initial infection, measles can exist permanently only where at least 250,000 people live in contact with each other.[10] That is the minimum number required to ensure that there will always be a sufficient number of uninfected individuals to keep a chain of infection going. Since most people who are not yet infected in such populations are children, measles is usually a childhood illness. When measles is introduced into isolated populations of less than 250,000 people, by contrast, the disease may sweep through not-previously-infected members of all ages, but then dies out until it is introduced again from outside.

Measles is widely regarded as a benign infection; for most persons infected, it is. However, for a minority, it may be deadly; measles kills about two million people a year worldwide, and between 1840 and 1990, killed about two hundred million.[11] The lethal potential of measles arises from two sources. First, measles cripples the body's immune system. In doing so, it is similar to the HIV virus that causes AIDS.[12] With the immune system impaired, other infectious agents can freely replicate, and this occurs even more rapidly in individuals who have poor nutrition or existing concurrent diseases. Thus, it is possible for individuals with measles to die from pneumonia, tuberculosis, typhoid, or other infections. This also explains why the mortality rate from measles may be as high as 10 percent in developing countries, compared to one-tenth of 1 percent in developed nations.

The other reason measles can be deadly is that it invades the brain. It apparently does this as a matter of course, since a study of electroencephalograms (EEGs) in children with uncomplicated measles showed that half of them had EEG changes.[13] In some individuals, the measles virus causes an acute or chronic infection of the brain (encephalitis). Before the introduction of measles vaccine in 1963, acute measles encephalitis affected approximately four thousand children in the United States each year, leaving one-quarter of them with deafness, blindness, seizures, mental retardation, or other brain damage.[14] In some cases, measles encephalitis may not become symptomatic for several years after the original infection and may then progress to coma and death.

The measles virus belongs to the morbillivirus family and is a direct offspring of the rinderpest virus of cattle. Studies of the molecular structure of measles virus have shown it to differ very little from its rinderpest parent and to be more closely related to rinderpest than are any of the other morbilliviruses.[15] Other members of the morbillivirus family that are more distantly related to the measles virus of humans are the canine distemper virus of dogs and other canines, pest-des-petits virus of sheep and goats, phocine distemper virus of seals, and distemper virus of dolphins.

The measles virus is thought to have evolved from the rinderpest virus after the domestication of cattle. Rinderpest is endemic in cattle and, when introduced to previously uninfected herds, can cause a severe epidemic. In the 1740s, rinderpest killed one-half of the cattle in France; in the 1890s, it devastated both cattle and related wild animals in Africa, as noted in chapter 1.

After humans domesticated animals, as we have seen, cattle and humans lived closely together; people milked their cows, helped them give birth, butchered them, and ate their meat. Drawings from Mesopotamia depict cows being milked, and paintings from ancient Egyptian tombs show different breeds of cattle. Until comparatively recently, in much of the world cattle and humans lived under the same roof; according to Thomas in *Man and the Natural World*, even in recent times in some areas of western Europe, it was said "that cows gave better milk if they could see the fire." Even people who themselves did not own cattle were exposed. "In the towns of the early modern period animals were everywhere, and the efforts of municipal authorities to prevent the inhabitants from keeping pigs or milking their cows in the street proved largely ineffective." [16]

Because the measles virus needs a population reservoir of at least 250,000 people to survive, measles as a disease did not exist before the rise of the urban centers in the Tigris-Euphrates, Nile, and Indus river valleys approximately five thousand years ago. Measles almost certainly existed after that time in the ancient world, but definitive descriptions are lacking because of its confusion with smallpox, chickenpox, rubella (German measles), scarlet fever, and other diseases that cause a rash. There are claims that measles was described in ancient Greece, Rome, Egypt, and China, but the first unequivocal description of the disease was provided by Al-Razi (Rhazes) in tenth-century Persia. This brilliant Muslim physician, whose full name was Abu Bakr Muhammad ibn Zakariyya of Ray, differentiated measles from smallpox and prescribed a treatment for both. Despite al-Razi's work, measles and smallpox continued to be confused for several hundred years more. However, by the seventeenth century, the two were definitely viewed as separate diseases, as illustrated by this quotation from English essayist Thomas Fuller: "Therefore the [measles] Pestilence can never breed the Small-Pox, nor the Small-Pox the Measles, . . . anymore than a Hen can a Duck, a Wolf a Sheep, or a Thistle Figs." [17]

"La Pequena Lepra"

The lethal potential of measles has been demonstrated many times in recent centuries when it has been introduced to previously unexposed populations. Mortality has been especially high in populations that suffer from poor nutrition and when measles has occurred in association with other diseases.

Since measles suppresses the immune system, any concurrent disease becomes more virulent.

A dramatic illustration of the effects of measles plus smallpox followed the arrival in the Americas of European explorers who inadvertently brought with them both viruses, along with other infectious diseases. Smallpox struck first and was rapidly followed by measles. For example, in 1529, "a measles epidemic in Cuba killed two-thirds of the natives who had survived smallpox."[18] In 1530, measles spread to Mexico and Peru, in 1531 to Honduras, and in 1532 to Nicaragua and Guatemala, killing up to half the inhabitants. A missionary wrote: "The Indians die so easily that the bare look and smell of a Spaniard caused them to give up the ghost."[19] Measles was known as "la pequena lepra" (the little leprosy) in contrast to "la gran lepra" of smallpox, which had preceded it.[20]

The devastation caused by these two diseases significantly altered the history of the New World. As noted by Karlen in *Man and Microbes:* "The toll of smallpox and measles was ten thousand here, a hundred thousand there, whole cities and tribes wiped out, cultures and languages lost. Corpses lay scattered in fields and heaped in silent villages."[21] Before the arrival of Europeans, the native populations of Mexico and Peru were between twenty-five and thirty million each; by the end of the sixteenth century, only approximately 10 percent of the population remained.[22] Confronted by the immunity of the Spaniards to these diseases (because they had been infected in childhood), the remaining natives accepted smallpox and measles as the white god's judgment on themselves and rapidly converted to Catholicism. The Aztec and Inca civilizations, among the most advanced in the world when the Europeans arrived, essentially ceased to exist as organized societies.

Elsewhere in the Americas, the effect of measles on the indigenous population was similar, if less well documented. In Florida, a measles epidemic in 1531 killed about half the native population; a second epidemic in 1596 killed one-quarter of those who remained.[23] In 1837, measles broke out on the North American plains among two thousand Mandan Indians who were under siege by their Sioux enemies. According to McNeil: "Their numbers were reduced from about 2,000 to a mere 30–40 survivors in a matter of weeks; and those survivors were promptly captured by enemies so that the Mandan tribe ceased to exist."[24] Canadian Indians similarly suffered. In 1819 and 1820, a measles epidemic killed "whole bands" of Chippewas; "one-third of the native population in the vicinity of Fort Chipewyan . . . is believed to have perished from an epidemic of dysentery accompanied by measles."[25]

The lethal effect of measles in combination with influenza was tragically illustrated when the two diseases simultaneously struck Alaska in 1900. According to studies of the epidemic, "a quarter of western Alaska's Eskimo population perished," with many villages virtually wiped out." At Ugavig, 60 of 132 inhabitants died. At Dog Fish Village on the Yukon River, 20 of 27 residents died. The Eskimos called it the "Great Sickness," and as a missionary described the epidemic: "Many were the wretched sights to be seen as the plague progressed. We used to go slopping along in the mud under a constant downpour of rain, through the stricken village of tents and cabins with our rumbling dead cart hauling out the unfortunate victims, while all around in the dark could be heard the fatal cough and groans of the sufferers. It was dismal work indeed. The very dogs ceased to howl, some forever, as the poor things overlooked in the general misery starved to death in their chains." And in another village: "At one place some passing strangers heard the crying of children, and upon examination found only some children left with both parents dead in the tent." [26]

On St. Paul Island, isolated in the Bering Sea, influenza arrived by ship on June 11, 1900. It infected virtually all the two hundred Aleut inhabitants and caused seven deaths. Two months later, measles arrived by another ship. It also infected virtually every inhabitant, so that "on 9 September only two Aleuts were not bedridden; . . . deaths continued almost daily until 3 October." Altogether, measles killed 10 percent of a population already weakened by influenza. [27]

There are many other examples of isolated human populations devastated by measles when initially exposed. In Iceland, an 1846 epidemic killed 2,026 people, 3 percent of the population. Another epidemic in 1882 killed 1,700 more. Measles first arrived in southern Greenland in 1951; out of a population of 4,262, all except 5 individuals were affected, and 77 died. [28]

In the South Pacific, measles arrived in then-isolated Sydney in 1834 and again in 1854, 1860, and 1867. The last epidemic was well documented; "in only a handful of months measles carried off more than 700 young children." This epidemic also illustrates the importance of poor nutrition and lower socioeconomic status as contributors to measles mortality. Among the poorest Sydney families, the mortality among children was approximately 30 percent, whereas among the wealthiest families, the mortality was less than 1 percent. [29]

Perhaps the best-known epidemic of measles swept through Fiji in 1875. The king of Fiji and his family had traveled to Australia to participate in the signing of a treaty with Britain, making Fiji a British colony. While in Australia, the king and his son were infected with measles, which was subsequently transmitted to other members of the group en route home. When the king arrived in Fiji, he was greeted by local chiefs, many of whom had traveled from the outer islands. Two days of discussions and celebrations followed, after which the chiefs returned home.

Within two months, measles had spread throughout Fiji, with lethal results. According to one account: "The attacks have been so sudden and complete that every soul in the village is down with it at once, and no one able to procure food or if procured cook it for themselves or others. . . . People have died of starvation and exhaustion in the midst of plenty."[30]

It was estimated that "not less than 40,000 Fijians died from the measles in the following four months out of a population of approximately 150,000, thus depleting the population by at least 27 percent."[31]

Among European settlers in the United States, measles was also a significant problem among rural populations that had not been exposed to the disease in childhood. During the Civil War, young men from rural areas were brought together with inevitable results: "Training programmes were so thoroughly disrupted by measles epidemics that companies, battalions and even whole regiments were disbanded temporarily and the men sent home."[32]

Knowledgeable Civil War commanders, aware that measles could devastate their troops, took only "seasoned" regiments into battle. When one Confederate general was asked to forward troops for battle, he promised to send them "as soon as [he could] have them put through the measles; a process which they are now undergoing—one-half of them now being sick." General Robert E. Lee also astutely noted the effects of measles on his troops: "We have a great deal of sickness among the soldiers, and now those on the sick-list would form an army. The measles is still among them, though I hope is dying out. But it is a disease which though light in childhood is severe in manhood, and prepares the system for other attacks. The constant rains, with no shelter but tents, have aggravated it."[33]

Measles favored neither side in the Civil War. Among Union forces, 76,318 cases, with 5,177 deaths, were recorded. At a Confederate camp in North Carolina, "4,000 cases of measles developed among 10,000 troops."[34]

The most famous Civil War victim of measles was, however, a fictional one. In Margaret Mitchell's novel *Gone with the Wind,* Scarlett O'Hara's first husband went off to war three weeks after their marriage. Less than two months later, Scarlett received a telegram informing her that her husband "had died ignominiously and swiftly of pneumonia, following measles, without ever having gotten any closer to the Yankees than the camp in South Carolina."[35]

Measles, then, is an example of a microbe that was originally transmitted from animals to humans but that became a problem only when humans came together in villages, towns, and urban centers. Other microbes also found urban living to their liking, spreading more easily from person to person. Some of the microbes became so successfully established in the new urban centers that they found new and even faster ways to spread themselves. Today Uruk and Thebes, tomorrow the world.

6

C H A P T E R

Humans as Traders

Microbes Get Passports

It is obvious that the equilibrium of human communities and of the animals kept by man has been drastically altered during the small number of generations since man was living as a highly successful nomadic predator animal. It is this disequilibrium which has imparted to infectious disease such an important role.

RICHARD FIENNES, Man, Nature, and Disease

For MILLIONS of years, microbes that were attached to mammals traveled neither very far nor very fast. Most hominids and other animals spent their lives in relatively circumscribed areas, and when they eventually migrated out of Africa, they traveled slowly. Since there were few opportunities for microbes to spread widely to nonimmune populations, microbe-caused disease epidemics were probably rare occurrences.

As Neolithic farmers settled into villages, and towns grew into urban centers, trade and warfare increased the opportunities for travel for humans, other animals, and the microbes that accompanied them. As early as nine thousand years ago, Catalahöyük in Turkey was a center of trade.

By the time the Mesopotamian civilizations flowered along the Tigris and Euphrates rivers, trading over long distances had become commonplace. Artisans of Mesopotamia produced pottery, leather goods, tools, and jewelry made from copper, silver, and gold, which were offered in trade. In exchange, Mesopotamians imported copper ore from Oman, gold and silver from Turkey, shells from India, lapis lazuli from Afghanistan, and cedar from Lebanon. Food was traded, including dates from Bahrain and wine from the shores of the Mediterranean. Domesticated animals were also commonly traded, and this was a major reason they spread so rapidly throughout the civilized world. The long-distance trade was often highly organized; 4,500 years ago, for example, Mesopotamia maintained a "colony" in Turkey to oversee its imports and exports.[1]

The speed with which humans, other animals, and microbes could travel increased substantially with the domestication of horses and camels and the introduction of ships. A journey that once had taken a week's walking could be completed in two days on horseback. At approximately the same time that horses were becoming widely used for travel, Egyptian merchant trading ships began plying the Mediterranean, later to be joined by Greek and Phoenician ships. From Lebanon came glass, textiles, metals, timber, and wine. From Egypt came linen, papyrus, gold, and ivory. From Cyprus came copper. From Arabia came dates, amber, and other resins. By the time of the Roman Empire, domesticated cattle were widely traded throughout the Near East and Europe, and Rome imported a thousand tons of wheat per day from North Africa.[2]

The movement of humans, domesticated animals, and microbes by trade routes was supplemented by warfare-associated travel. Disputes between neighboring groups of hominids had certainly always existed, but horses and ships elevated sporadic fighting to the level of warfare. Sargon the Great led military campaigns from Mesopotamia into Syria and Turkey more than four thousand years ago; five hundred years later, Persians invaded and destroyed the cities of the Indus Valley in Pakistan. When chariots were invented and attached to horses approximately four thousand years ago, power shifted to the Hittites and other horse-raising groups from the Asian steppes.

With the use of camels, horses, and ships, the pace of the world accelerated. Along established trade routes, increasing numbers of people, animals, and microbes interacted with each other in crowded bazaars and caravansaries. Warfare brought famine, rape, and the forcible resettlement of large numbers of slaves and animals as spoils of war. Before the introduction of ships, "dispersal of disease over long distances was slow and required a larger host population to remain intact until it reached a new population," but with ships the passengers "could act as a disease reservoir with reasonably swift dispersal" of the disease."[3] Bacteria, viruses, and protozoa that had remained relatively localized for millions of years found themselves in new environments and in contact with large numbers of susceptible humans and other animals.

The consequences of this unprecedented human movement were predictable. Ancient heirloom infections like hepatitis, malaria, and yellow fever and more recent diseases like measles, smallpox, and tuberculosis, which had come from animal domestication, began spreading more widely. Epidemics followed.

The first suggestion of epidemics in human history comes from Mesopotamia, where there is "a stone inscription describing epidemics and invoking the Goddess of Epidemics."[4] Among these are the biblical "ten plagues" that led to the release of the Hebrews from their Egyptian enslavement; a "pestilence" that killed 70,000 Israelis in three days;[5] and a disease said to have killed 185,000 Assyrians overnight.[6]

Epidemics were also recorded by the ancient Greek writers. The most noteworthy, as we will see in chapter 11, was the plague of Athens, which reached its height around 430 B.C.E. The epidemic was thought to have arisen in Ethiopia and to have affected Egypt before moving to the port of Piraeus and then to the rest of the Athens city-state. Recent excavations carried out during the building of the Athens subway confirmed the existence of the plague: A mass grave was uncovered that contained the remains of many plague victims, who had apparently been buried in great haste.[7] This discovery appears to confirm the observation of Thucydides, who wrote: "All the funeral ceremonies which used to be observed were now disorganized, and they buried the dead as best they could. Many people, lacking the necessary means of burial because so many deaths had already occurred in their households, adopted the most shameless methods."[8] The cause of the plague in Athens has been the subject of intense speculation but has never been conclusively identified. However, the effects of the plague are clear: It resulted in the death of approximately one-third of the population of Athens.

Even allowing for an apocryphal element in some of these accounts, it seems evident that epidemics of disease periodically swept the Middle East and eastern Mediterranean region in an era in which human travel was increasing, both in numbers and speed. Medical speculations have been legion regarding which human disease caused which ancient epidemic. The results are quite unsatisfactory because the descriptions of most of these epidemics are too fragmentary to allow for specific attribution. Among diseases that have been suggested are measles, smallpox, influenza, typhoid, typhus, glanders, and plague. The last is least likely since rats, which carry plague, had not yet arrived in the Middle East.

The Arrival of Rats

Mice and rats are rodents, along with squirrels, chipmunks, marmots, gerbils, hamsters, guinea pigs, woodchucks, beavers, and porcupines. Mice and rats originally evolved in central Asia, India, and Pakistan and were confined to that region for millions of years. At Bhimbetka in northern India, there is an ancient but undated rock drawing of several rats being carried in a bag.

Mice and rats diverged approximately ten million years ago; DNA differences between them, in fact, are ten times greater than DNA differences between chimpanzees and humans.[9]

Rats migrated from their ancient homeland rather late in history. The Greeks and Romans had no word for them, and, according to Hans Zinsser's *Rats, Lice, and History,* "most scholars agree that there is no reliable mention of rats — as such — in classical literature."[10] When the rats finally did migrate, they carried with them *Yersinia pestis,* the bacteria that causes human plague. Plague is transmitted from rats to humans by using fleas as vectors; the fleas bite infected rats, then bite humans, and thereby transmit the bacteria.

Yersinia pestis is unusual insofar as it is, in microbial terms, a relative newcomer. It evolved from, and is almost identical to, *Yersinia pseudotuberculosis,* a bacteria that is widely distributed among rodents, other mammals, and birds. In humans, *Yersinia pseudotuberculosis* causes a mild intestinal disease. According to recent molecular studies, *Yersinia pestis* evolved from *Yersinia pseudotuberculosis* sometime within the past few thousand years, "shortly before the first known pandemics of human plague."[11]

What causes a comparatively harmless bacteria like *Yersinia pseudotuberculosis* to undergo changes in genetic structure and evolve into a closely related but highly malignant *Yersinia pestis?* Such changes may occur when a bacteria infects an animal species it has not previously infected. They may also occur when two different microbes infect a single mammal at the same time, resulting in an exchange of genetic material between the microbes. This is the same mechanism that makes some strains of influenza so deadly, as we will see in chapter 9. There is some evidence that *Yersinia pseudotuberculosis* may have undergone malignant transformation as part of a simultaneous infection of a mammal with *Salmonella typhi,* a related bacteria that causes typhoid fever.[12] The transformation of *Yersinia pseudotuberculosis* into the plague bacteria almost certainly took place in central Asia, since *Yersinia pestis* even today is endemic among marmots and gerbils of that region; it does not cause apparent disease in them, although it does cause disease in rats. The transformation to *Yersinia pestis* may therefore have occurred when *Yersinia pseudotuberculosis* made the jump from marmots and gerbils to rats.

The evolution of one species of bacteria into a closely related species with different properties presumably occurs frequently in nature. In the case of *Yersinia pestis,* we would not even be aware of its existence had it remained a microbe of rodents living remotely from humans, as rats once did. However, once humans began to travel, rats traveled with them. Rats joined caravans of traders going back and forth between the Middle East and China, passing directly through the rats' ancient homeland. And rats in large numbers came aboard ships and traveled by sea. The most common rat at that time was the black rat (*Rattus rattus*), originally a tree dweller known for its remarkable climbing ability. It is said to easily climb up "slick-painted drainpipes, elevator cables, or telephone wires" and "can gnaw a hole in a ceiling while at the same time gripping tightly an electric wire."[13] The black rat thus had no difficulty entering and exiting ships on mooring lines. As trade increased, so did the distribution of the black rat.

Once rats arrived in a new area or disembarked at a new port, they spread rapidly because they are so prolific. They can breed at four to six months of age, have a gestation period of only twenty days, and have four or five litters each year, with up to ten rat pups in each litter. By one estimate, a single rat can theoretically produce as many as fifteen thousand descendents in a year.[14] This rapid rate of reproduction also means, in evolutionary terms, that rats can quickly adapt to new conditions and climates.

The first definite appearance of rats in the Mediterranean region was not until the sixth century C.E. The rats, infected with *Yersinia pestis*, probably arrived by ship, since plague first appeared in port cities of Egypt. From there, it spread quickly to Constantinople, where "panic, disorder, and murder reigned in the streets. . . . There were too many corpses to bury. The roofs were removed from the city's fortified towers, and bodies were stacked in them like cordwood. Soon the towers filled, and the stench became unbearable. People kept dying, up to 10,000 each day, and there was no place to put the corpses. Rafts were loaded with the dead, rowed out to sea, and set adrift. When this bout of plague ended, 40 percent of the city's people had died."[15] Contemporary descriptions leave little doubt about the diagnosis: "They had a sudden fever; . . . not many days after, a bubonic swelling developed. . . . With some the body broke out in black postules . . . and these did not survive even one day."[16] The swellings, or bubos, were enlarged lymph nodes and are characteristic of plague.

This was the plague of Justinian, named after the emperor of the eastern Roman Empire who ruled from Constantinople.

The Black Death

In the centuries following the plague of Justinian in the sixth century C.E., periodic outbreaks recurred but on a smaller scale. The black rat continued to spread by land and by sea, increasing significantly in Europe with the returning Crusaders. When rats reached Ireland, the Irish called them "French mice."[17] By the thirteenth century, rats had become so abundant that they threatened food supplies.

In central Germany, the town of Hamelin was infested. According to legend, a mysterious piper appeared and offered to rid the town of rats for a certain sum. The townspeople accepted the proposal, and the piper thereupon played his pipe and led the rats into the Weser River, where they drowned. When the town refused to pay him, the piper returned the next day, played his pipe again, and this time led the town's children to a mountain cave, where all but two disappeared.

By the fifteenth century, rat catchers had become valued citizens in Europe and were organized into guilds. In some areas, they wore multicolored (pied) uniforms and carried flags with pictures of rats on them. Some rat catchers became wealthy, since they were paid a bounty for each rat they caught; in addition, rat skins were used to make inexpensive coats, gloves, and trim for collars. Shakespeare alludes to rats several times, as when Hamlet plunges his sword through a drapery, thinking that Claudius hides there, and cries: "How now! A rat? Dead, for a ducat, dead!"[18] It was also at this time that Cervantes wrote in *Don Quixote de la Mancha*: "I begin to smell a rat."[19] In later centuries, rat catchers were immortalized in literature, as in Goethe's poem "The Rat Catcher," and in paintings by Vischer and Rembrandt.

The Black Death, or Great Pestilence as it was known at the time, began in 1338 at Issyk Kul, in what is now Krygyzstan in central Asia. Plague broke out in a trading community and spread south into India, east into China, and west toward the Middle East along the caravan routes. By 1346, it had reached the shores of the Mediterranean and Black seas. In Aleppo and Gaza, five hundred people died each day, and rumors reached Europe that "all of India was said to be depopulated, whole territories covered by dead bodies, other areas with no one left alive."[20]

On April 27, 1348, three ships arrived in Genoa from Caffa, a major Genoese trading port on the Black Sea (now Feodosiya, Ukraine). According to a contemporary writer, the ships were "carrying horrible disease from the East."[21] Simon Boccanegra, the Genoese doge who would later be immortalized by a Verdi opera, turned the ships away. Another ship from Caffa arrived in Messina, Sicily, "with dead and dying men at the oars."[22] Soon the plague had swept ashore at every Mediterranean port, carried by the fleas on the dying rats and men.

In contrast to the sixth-century plague, the fourteenth-century plague spread throughout Europe because black rats had by then become widespread. A favorite place for them to live was in the thatch roofs of dwellings used by all except the wealthiest people. When rats died, their infected fleas dropped onto the people who lived below. As has been noted, "the distribution and density of the rat population governs the distribution and intensity of the human disease."[23] Carried by ships, plague spread up the Arno to Florence and up the Rhone to Avignon; then it continued inland.

Italy, with three of the four largest cities in Europe, was hardest hit. Siena, Parma, Verona, Genoa, and Naples lost half their populations. Giovanni Boccaccio in his 1353 *Decameron* described the plague in Florence:

> Many dropped dead in the open streets, both by day and by night, whilst a great many others, though dying in their own houses, drew their neighbors' attention to the fact more by the smell of their rotting corpses than by any other means. And what with these, and the others dying all over the city, bodies were here, there and everywhere. . . . Tedious were it to recount, how citizen avoided citizen, how among neighbors was scarce found any that shewed fellow-feeling for another, how kinsfolk held aloof, and never met, or but rarely; enough that this sore affliction entered so deep into the minds of men and women, that in the horror thereof brother was forsaken by brother, nephew by uncle, brother by sister, and oftentimes husband by wife: nay, what is more, and scarcely to be believed, fathers and mothers were found to abandon their own children, untended, unvisited, to their fate, as if they had been strangers. . . . It was come to this, that a dead man was then of no more account than a dead goat would be today.[24]

Italian poet Francesco Petrarch, whose beloved Laura died from the plague, asked: "Is it possible that posterity can believe these things? For we, who have seen them, can hardly believe them."[25]

At Avignon in southern France, when graveyards filled up, bodies "were thrown into the Rhone until mass burial pits were dug for dumping the corpses."[26] Avignon was the seat of the papacy from 1309 to 1377, and Pope Clement VI, on orders of his physicians, sat quietly between two huge blazing fireplaces until the plague had passed. King Philip VI asked the medical faculty at the University of Paris what was causing the plague; they replied that it was caused by an unusual alignment of the planets, and this belief became widespread. In many French, Swiss, and German cities, Jews were blamed for the plague and were persecuted; in Strasbourg, an estimated nine hundred Jews were burned to death on February 14, 1349.[27]

Month after month, the Great Pestilence rolled northward into England, Ireland, Scotland, and Scandinavia, eventually reaching even Iceland and Greenland. Off the coast of Norway, a ship ran aground because its entire crew had died.[28] Monasteries, hospitals, and prisons, where many people lived closely together, were especially affected, since infected fleas could move quickly among their inhabitants. In Montpellier in France, only 7 of 140 Dominicans survived.[29] At a monastery at Ivy Church in England, only 1 of 13 monks lived.[30] And at a monastery in Kilkenny, Ireland, a monk watched each of his brothers die until he was the only one left. Before he, too, died, he wrote:

> Now I, brother John Clyn, of the Order of Minor Friars and the commu-
> nity of Kilkenny, have written in this book these notable events that have
> occurred in my time, which I have learned from the evidence of my own
> eyes or upon reliable report. And lest [these] notable events should per-
> ish with time and fade from the memory of future generations, . . . while
> waiting among the dead for the coming of death, I have set them down
> in writing just as I have truthfully heard and examined them. And lest the
> writing should perish with the writer and the work with the workman, I
> leave the parchment for the work to be continued in case in the future
> any human survivor should remain, or someone of the race of Adam
> should be able to escape this plague and continue what I have begun.[31]

In these small communities, it must have seemed as if the end of the world
had truly arrived.

Historians disagree regarding the number of people who died during the
Great Pestilence from 1348 to 1350, with most estimates ranging from one-
quarter to one-third of Europe's population. There are also disagreements regarding the relative role of other diseases, especially anthrax and typhus, in
increasing the mortality. It seems certain, however, that plague was the main
cause of death, since there are many classic descriptions of the symptoms,
especially enlarged lymph nodes (bubos) in the groin or armpit, depending
on whether the initial fleabite was on the person's leg or arm.

The effect of the Great Pestilence on European society was profound.
Norman Cantor called it "the greatest biomedical disaster in European and
possibly in world history" and discussed at length the social and economic
disruption it brought about.[32] A shortage of labor led directly to the Peasants'
Revolt of 1381 and the subsequent decline of serfdom. The fact that a dispro-
portionate number of monks and priests died undermined the Church; if this
was God's will, he was indeed a mysterious God. The plague also provided
impetus to the development of public health, since it was the first time that
quarantines were used; arriving ships were forced to lie at anchor for forty
days (*quarant* is the French word for "forty") until it was certain there was no
plague on board.

During the 1350s, the Great Pestilence slowly diminished, but smaller
epidemics of plague continued to recur in Europe and throughout the world.
Outbreaks in Venice between 1575 and 1577 and again from 1630 to 1631
are said to have killed one-third of the population. England had major outbreaks in 1563, 1593, 1603, and 1625, but these were eclipsed by the Great
Plague of London in 1665, when half the population, including King Charles
II and his entire court, fled the city. Of those who remained, approximately
one-third died. This outbreak of plague was noteworthy in being documented
by Samuel Pepys in his *Diary* and later fictionalized by Daniel Defoe in his

Journal of the Plague Year. The Great Plague of London was also memorable because of widespread beliefs that venereal disease and smoking provided some immunity from the plague. It has been speculated that "the modern use of tobacco in Britain . . . may have derived from its supposititious efficacy as a prophylactic against bubonic plague, for the menace of plague and the terror inspired by its rumored approach persisted among the population until late in the nineteenth century."[33] Strong odors were also believed to be protective and gave rise to the wearing of eau de cologne, based on an eighteenth-century formula from Cologne, Germany, among those who could afford it.

Plague in the United States

Plague entered the United States on January 2, 1900, by way of infected rats on a steamship that arrived in San Francisco. The ship had come from Honolulu, which, along with Hong Kong, Kobe, and other Pacific ports, was experiencing plague.

The 1900 epidemic had begun in 1894 in central Asia. A change in women's fashions had made the fur of marmots more valuable, so Manchurian hunters began trapping and selling them.[34] Since *Yersinia pestis* is widespread among marmots, some of the hunters contracted plague. It spread to Hong Kong, and then in 1896 to India.

San Francisco's first deaths occurred in Chinatown, adjacent to the docks. The year 1900 was, ironically, the Year of the Rat on the Chinese calendar. Over the following eight years, 280 San Francisco residents were infected with plague, with 172 reported deaths.[35] It was suspected that others died, but many Chinese families surreptitiously buried their dead so that the bodies would not be desecrated by autopsy. The main reason mortality was not greater was that a French bacteriologist, Alexandre Yersin, had identified the bacteria that caused the disease and correctly surmised that it was being spread by rats. Therefore, public health authorities in San Francisco implemented a campaign to kill the city's rats.

That Chinese immigrants made up the majority of people affected by the plague in San Francisco (because they lived closest to its point of origin) led to anti-Chinese sentiment. It fed a growing xenophobia among white Americans, who feared that immigrants from foreign countries were bringing diseases with them. A similar anti-Jewish sentiment arose in Baltimore in the late nineteenth century following a cholera epidemic in which poor Jewish immigrants were severely affected. This association of immigrants with infectious diseases was a major impetus to the immigration restriction movement, culminating in the Immigration Restriction Act of 1921, which established quotas of immigrants by country of origin, and subsequently to the Johnson-Reed Act of 1924, which virtually abolished immigration from some nations.

By the time plague had come under control in San Francisco in 1908, *Yersinia pestis* had spread beyond the city. Rats carried it across the bay to Oakland, and from there it moved into the countryside, infecting squirrels, chipmunks, prairie dogs, and other rodents. During the twentieth century, plague moved slowly but progressively eastward, so that by the end of the century, it had been reported in rodents in the Dakotas, Nebraska, Kansas, Oklahoma, and Texas.[36] There is no reason to believe that this eastward march is not continuing.

Presently, there are only approximately ten reported human cases of plague each year in the United States, with most occurring in California, Arizona, New Mexico, and Colorado. In 2002, a couple from New Mexico who were visiting New York City were diagnosed with plague, setting off fears of terrorism.[37] The fears proved unfounded but were based on the fact that plague can be spread by droplets as well as by fleas; thus, aerosolized, it is a potential agent for use by bioterrorists. So traumatic was the news of the two cases of plague in New York that the *New York Times* on November 8, 2002, felt the need to publish an editorial reassuring people that "we have antibiotics to quell the germ, and good supportive care."

What is the future of plague? Since the disease is permanently established in rats and other rodents throughout the world, its eradication is out of the question.

Rats are extremely hardy, with the brown rat (*Rattus Norvegicus*), which became widespread in the eighteenth century, even more difficult to exterminate than the black rat (*Rattus rattus*). Brown rats are excellent swimmers; they can "tread water for three days, . . . survive being flushed down a toilet and have been found alive in a block of ice." Both black rats and brown rats can also "chew through metal, wood and concrete" with their sharp incisors.[38] In many cities, black and brown rats coexist; both can be affected by, and thus carry, the plague.

Periodic outbreaks of plague should therefore be expected. In 2003, for example, an outbreak of plague affected eleven people in Oran, Algeria;[39] ironically, this city was the setting for Albert Camus's *The Plague*, a fictional account of such an epidemic.

In the United States, conditions favorable to plague exist in many cities. Even in affluent Beverly Hills, for example, rats have become abundant, using the city's "fruit trees, bird feeders, swimming pools and dog-food bowls." According to a news story in September 2002, "over the past two months a half dozen restaurants have temporarily closed along Santa Monica Promenade because of rats" and a "well-to-do doctor . . . found five rats swimming in his marble pool on a recent Saturday afternoon."[40] In New York City, there are an estimated twelve rats for every person;[41] the city's Department of Health has posted on its Web page the symptoms of plague and its proper treatment.[42] *Yersinia pestis* could arrive in eastern port cities by ship, or eventually by its continuing spread across the country, carried by squirrels, prairie dogs, and other rodents.

The immediate threat of a plague epidemic in the United States is minimal because the plague bacteria continues to be sensitive to some antibiotics. As long as antibiotics are started early in the course of illness, anyone infected with plague should recover. If, on the other hand, *Yersinia pestis* should mutate either through natural evolution or by terrorism-related modifications, it could become antibiotic resistant. Plague could again become not just a fatal disease but a synonym for disaster.

Mice and Hantavirus Infection

In contrast to rats, mice migrated out of central Asia much earlier in human history. By the time Neolithic farmers began settling in permanent dwellings approximately ten thousand years ago, four species of mice had already spread to the Middle East and North Africa.[43] One of these, the common house mouse (*Mus musculus*) moved into dwellings and became humans' first houseguest. Thus, it is not surprising that mice are described in the Old Testament and were well known to the Greeks and Romans.

As humans spread around the world, mice accompanied them. And like all animals, mice brought along their microbes. Hantaviruses are microbes carried by many species of mice, rats, voles, and other rodents. The hantaviruses and rodents have adapted to each other over millions of years, so the microbes cause no apparent illness in the rodents. A recent summary of these viruses notes that "each virus has adapted to a single or a small group of rodent hosts with which it has a commensal relationship, being transmitted from adults to young animals and causing lifelong persistent infections."[44] As part of this lifelong infection, hantaviruses are chronically shed in the rodents' saliva, urine, and feces.

The importance of rodent-carried hantaviruses became clear during the Korean War. Over 3,000 UN troops developed Korean hemorrhagic fever; more than 300 died, including 121 Americans. It was eventually shown that the disease was caused by a hantavirus carried by a Korean field mouse, and it is thought that the troops had been exposed by sleeping on the ground in areas with large numbers of mice.

Hantaviruses became prominent in the United States in 1993, with an outbreak of hantavirus pulmonary syndrome among young adults in the Four Corners area of the Southwest. Within two weeks, nineteen individuals were affected, twelve of whom died. The disease begins with fever, headache, muscle aches, and a cough. The lungs are primarily affected, and death can come quickly if the lungs fill with fluid. Since the disease was first recognized in 1993, 353 cases have been reported in the United States, including 132 deaths.[45]

The virus that has caused most cases of hantavirus pulmonary syndrome in the United States is carried by deer mice and has been designated the *Sin Nombre* (without a name) virus. Studies have shown that approximately 10 percent of deer mice shed the virus, which may then become airborne in microscopic particles when, for example, a person sweeps up mouse droppings.[46] Exposure to deer mice and their droppings has been a common denominator in most cases of hantavirus pulmonary syndrome caused by *Sin Nombre* virus.

Since the *Sin Nombre* virus has infected mice for millions of years, it has presumably caused occasional past cases of human disease but was not recognized as such. Why, then, did it become visible in the United States only in 1993?

The primary reason for the outbreak in 1993 was ecological. The southwestern United States experienced a severe drought in the years that preceded 1992, then had abundant precipitation during the winter of 1992–1993. This led to a record number of wild piñon nuts, which deer mice eat, in the spring of 1993. The deer mice, therefore, proliferated rapidly, increasing tenfold between 1992 and 1993.[47] And when the piñon nuts ran out, the mice invaded the dwellings of people who lived in the area, thus exposing many more people to the virus than would have been exposed under normal climatic conditions.

The *Sin Nombre* hantavirus disease outbreak has focused attention on hantaviruses in general. At least seventeen different hantaviruses have been identified, nine of which are found in the United States. Each is adapted to one or more rodents, and their potential for causing human diseases is under investigation.

The hantavirus disease outbreak has also served as an unpleasant reminder that animals carry thousands of microbes currently unknown to us. When ecological conditions change, either naturally or through human intervention, such microbes may produce outbreaks of diseases not previously recognized.

CHAPTER

Humans as Pet Keepers

Microbes Move into the Bedroom

> *Our domesticated animals have become less an integral part of our*
> *struggle for survival and more surrogates in our need for social fulfillment.*
> *As such, they become even more intimately part of our extended families.*
> *They enjoy our medical system and become potential vectors of pathogens*
> *at levels previously known only in members of our own species.*
>
> LARRY MARTIN, "Earth History"

DURING the ten thousand years since humans began domesticating animals, we have kept them primarily to supply our material needs. Their meat, milk, and eggs have been our major source of protein; their wool, skins, and fur have been our most important sources of clothing; and until the invention of the gasoline-powered engine, they were the main source of transportation for people and goods. They have also helped plow fields, herd sheep, turn waterwheels, guard the home, protect grain supplies from rodents, and track wild animals during the hunt. By supplying our material needs, animals have played a critical role in advancing human civilization.

Using animals to supply our emotional needs, by contrast, is relatively new. The keeping of pets has always existed on a small scale but has been widespread for only the past three hundred years and especially prominent in Western culture for only the past fifty years. This is bringing about a fundamental change in the way humans and other animals interact and exchange microbes.

Occasional pet keeping probably dates to the time when Paleolithic hunters brought home infant offspring of their kill as curiosities or playthings for their children. Twentieth-century anthropological accounts of remaining

68

hunter-gatherer societies include descriptions of such pet keeping. Ancient Egyptians also were enthusiastic pet keepers, especially families in the upper classes. Some dogs wore collars with names inscribed, such as "Ebony" or "Cooking-Pot."[1] Cats, known in Egyptian as "miu," were associated with the goddess of fertility, and, according to one historian, by the fourth century B.C.E., "the status of cats . . . seems to have been roughly equivalent to that of cows in present day India. Many people owned pet cats, and the death of one sent the entire family into mourning, shaving their eyebrows as a mark of respect."[2]

Pet keeping among the aristocracy has been widespread over the centuries. As James Serpell noted in his *In the Company of Animals:* "Throughout history the world's ruling classes have almost invariably demonstrated a powerful affinity for pets, and this affinity has often been the excuse for mind-boggling displays of gratuitous self-indulgence." As examples, Serpell cites the Roman emperor Hadrian, who had "monumental tombstones erected over the graves of his favorite dogs"; the Han Chinese emperor Ling, who gave his dogs "the rank of senior court officials . . . and a personal bodyguard of hand-picked soldiers"; and the Japanese shogun Tsunayoshi, who owned a hundred thousand dogs and "passed a law that all dogs must be treated kindly and only spoken to in the politest of terms."[3]

Pet keeping by aristocrats was also popular in mediaeval Europe. According to sociologist Joanna Swabe: "From the late middle ages onwards, the practice of keeping 'toy' dogs became increasingly fashionable in aristocratic circles. . . . Mediaeval noble women, for example, were inclined to carry such dogs around with them and feed them scraps from the table. . . . By the sixteenth century, the practice of keeping lap-dogs had become extremely popular within English high society." One writer chastised "these kind of people, who delight more in dogs that are deprived of all possibility of reason, than they do in children that be capable of wisdom and judgment."[4]

The status of pets among the English aristocracy reached its apogee in the early seventeenth century. James I, who became king in 1603, kept many pet dogs and "was accused in 1617 of loving his dogs more than his subjects."[5] His ill-fated mother, Mary Queen of Scots, was also fond of dogs. Reportedly, following her execution, her headless body was seen to move, causing great consternation among those gathered to witness the event. This movement was found to have been caused by her little dog, which, unknown to her executioners, had been resting beneath her capacious clothing.

Elizabeth, daughter of James I, "was notorious for preferring her pets to her children." James's son, Charles I, who ascended to the throne in 1625, "only parted with his own dog after receiving sentence of death in 1649," and his son, Charles II, "was notorious for playing with his dog at the Council table." Aristocrats of the era emulated the royal family, so that "hounds were often better fed than the servants, and they were sometimes better housed."[6] But the popularity of dogs as pets did not extend to the middle or lower classes. Shakespeare usually referred to dogs in derogatory terms as, for example, "whoreson dog," "thou damn'd, inexecrable dog," and "you bawling, blasphemous, incharitable dog."[7] Thomas Brooks in 1662 referred to dogs as "vermin," and in paintings of this period dogs often symbolized "gluttony, lust, coarse bodily functions and general disruptiveness."[8]

The Rise of Dogs and Cats

Dogs and cats are the most popular pets in most parts of the world today. Both animals are a manageable size, relatively easy to maintain and train, playful, and seemingly intelligent. Also, as noted by Joanna Swabe, "both species are particularly communicative and possess an extensive range of facial expressions, typical body and tail postures, sounds and so forth that humans believe they can understand."[9]

In seventeenth-century Europe, the keeping of pet dogs began to slowly spread from the aristocracy to the middle class. Dogs were increasingly given personal names, allowed in the home, and even taken to church, where large dogs could function as foot warmers.[10]

One measure of the increase in dogs as pets is the number of breeds available. All dogs are descended from the common wolf; different breeds develop as the result of selective breeding of dogs with unusual physical characteristics caused by mutations, such as a curly tail or long hair, or specific behavioral traits, such as the ability to herd sheep. In 1800 in England, there were only fifteen breeds of dogs; by 1900 the number had increased to sixty, and by the year 2000, to more than four hundred.[11] Pet dogs had become so common in France by the mid–nineteenth century that the government put a tax on nonworking dogs; at that time, there were one hundred thousand dogs in Paris alone. By the end of the nineteenth century, dog-care books had become widely available, dog shows were becoming popular, and a pet cemetery had opened in Paris, guaranteeing for fifty francs a private plot for the deceased dog for ten years.[12]

Cats, by contrast, became popular as pets much more slowly. In the ancient world, they had been kept as pets in Egypt and possibly Cyprus, but elsewhere until the eighteenth century, people used cats to control rodents but rarely viewed them as pets. During the Middle Ages, they were associated with witches and Satan, both of which were believed capable of transforming themselves into cats. Witches were also thought to ride on the backs of giant cats to their nocturnal Sabbats, where they participated in orgies with demons and devils. As these beliefs became widespread, people treated cats with increasing cruelty, especially on Christian holidays. "Lent was a particularly hard time for medieval cats. They were killed and buried in Oldenburg, Westphalia, Belgium, Switzerland and Bohemia; burnt on Shrove Tuesday in the Vosges, and in Alsace at Easter. In the Ardennes they were thrown into bonfires or roasted in the ends of long poles, or in wicker baskets on the first Sunday in Lent."[13]

Keeping cats as pets began among writers and intellectuals in eighteenth-century England and France. In England, Samuel Johnson kept a pet cat, Thomas Gray wrote an "Ode on the Death of a Favorite Cat, Drowned in a Tub of Gold Fishes," and Christopher Smart, in his poem "On Jeoffry, My Cat," praised his cat as "the servant of the Living God, duly and daily serving him." In France, novelist Francois Chateaubriand wrote: "What I like about the cat is his character, independent and almost heartless. . . . The cat lives alone, he has no need of society." Chateaubriand especially admired the cat for "that indifference with which he passes from salon to gutter," according to Kathleen Kete's *The Beast in the Boudoir*. The cat, Kete observes, "became a trope of intellectuals, . . . a sign for the literary life, a signature."[14] By the end of the eighteenth century, cats had achieved some gentility, so that in 1792, a Mrs. Griggs in London reportedly "bequested £150 per annum so that a trusted black servant could continue to care for her eighty-six cats."[15]

The association of pet cats with writers and intellectuals continued well into the nineteenth century. In England, Shelley and Wordsworth wrote lovingly of cats; in France, Baudelaire, in his poem "The Cat," merged the animal with his mistress;[16] and in America, Poe wrote with his pet tortoiseshell perched upon his shoulder. By that time, cats were more widely accepted as pets and had become associated with children. A French writer noted that "the cat is the nurse's favorite and the baby's earliest friend."[17] An 1836 U.S. essay described children at play, "dressing themselves, or perhaps a favorite dog or kitten, in the most ludicrous and fanciful attire."[18] And cats took their place in nursery rhymes:

> *Great A, little A, bouncing B,*
> *Cat's in the cupboard, and can't see me.*

In the latter half of the nineteenth century, the keeping of cats as pets increased markedly, and for the first time they began to challenge dogs in popularity. Advertisers used cats extensively to attract attention to their products, including "soap, thread boxes, games, hosiery, stove cleaner, shoe polish, rat poison, oils and cigar boxes." Among the last, cigars with the Me-ow label first appeared in 1886, Tabby cigars in 1894, White Cat in 1908, and Pussy in 1910. In 1914,

Kellogg's advertised cornflakes with a picture of a young girl eating her cereal while holding her cat; the accompanying slogan read: "For Kiddies, Not Kitties." Procter and Gamble advertised Ivory soap with a picture of twelve black cats and one white cat and the slogan "Ivory Soap: 99 and 44/100 percent pure."[19] The use of black cats in advertising was especially eye-catching, since they had been viewed for centuries as symbols of witchcraft.

The increasing acceptance of cats as pets can also be measured by their presence in art. Before 1700, cats were depicted only rarely in paintings and, when included, usually represented malevolent forces. An example is Lorenzo Lotto's "Annunciation," painted in 1534, which shows an angel announcing the coming Christ child and a cat running away from the angel, indicating the banishment of evil. In the eighteenth century, cats were occasionally included in paintings, and in the nineteenth century they became commonplace, as, for example, in two Renoir paintings of young women holding cats.

By the end of the nineteenth century, then, dogs and cats had both become firmly established as pets in Western cultures. In England, "domestic animals added to the comfort of the home," while in France "bourgeois Parisians insistently associated petkeeping with modernity."[20] The first cat show was held in London's Crystal Palace in 1871, and by the end of the century such shows had spread throughout Europe and America. An 1892 article in the *Atlantic Monthly* illustrates how far cats had come from being burned as Lenten offerings: "Of late years there has been a rapid and promising growth of what disaffected and alliterative critics call the 'cat cult,' and poets and painters vie with one another in celebrating the charms of this long-neglected pet."[21]

Contemporary Pet Keeping

The increase in pet keeping in the past half century is unique in human history. In the United States and Europe, more than half of all homes have one household animal and a substantial number have several. U.S. homes have an estimated 55 million dogs, 64 million cats, 31 million caged birds, 7 million reptiles, 87 million aquarium fish, and more than 12 million other "small animals."[22] American dogs are said to annually deposit two million tons of feces on streets, in yards, and sometimes in homes. In the Netherlands, it has been estimated that "cats produce 100,000 tons of waste per annum," and cat litter "makes up five per cent of Dutch refuse."[23]

Pet keeping may still be on the increase. Between 1994 and 1998, for example, the sale of cat food rose 11 percent in both the United States and western Europe. The two largest U.S. suppliers of pet food and pet accessories, PETsMART and Petco, reported increased sales of 8 and 11 percent, respectively, in 2002, and Petco announced that it planned to add sixty new stores to the six hundred it already owned.[24]

In other parts of the world, pet keeping is growing even faster. Between 1994 and 1998, cat-food sales rose by 20 percent in Asia and 48 percent in Latin America.[25] As the middle class expands in many developing countries, pet ownership is increasing proportionately. Even China, where pets have been considered bourgeois and "running dog" has been a popular expletive, is experiencing a "boom in pet ownership." Pet dogs and cats are the newest Chinese symbol of success, and it has been projected "that China in 2050 will have more than 500 million cats and dogs."[26]

Numbers, however, reveal only part of this contemporary change in animal-human relationships. Equally important is the increased contact, and indeed intimacy, between humans and their pet animals. Many pets, especially dogs and cats, are increasingly considered family members and cared for almost as if they were human. We indulge pets today in ways that would have been unimaginable in past years.

For example, a 1999 poll of pet owners reported that 16 percent of household dogs sleep on top of their owner's bed, and an additional 2 percent sleep in the bed. The same survey reported that "67 percent of America's cats are allowed to sleep on their owner's beds or anywhere they want"; in a 2003 survey of cat owners, 75 percent answered "frequently" when asked how often they "kiss the cat or allow it to lick you"; and 11 percent of dog owners "say they feel closest to their pets while exchanging kisses."[27]

The increasing intimacy between pet owners and their pets reflects pets having become members of the family. As one pet owner explained: "When I was growing up, a dog was just an add-on to the family, but it really wasn't like a person. But now, with many people, dogs have become much more like a member of the family." That pets have become family members is also suggested by the 58 percent of pet owners who include their pet in family or holiday portraits, the 55 percent who call themselves their pet's "mom" or "dad," and the 39 percent who "have more pictures of their pets than of their spouse or significant other."[28]

The close relationship between pets and their owners also shows up in the number of pets that owners take along on trips. One survey reported that "nearly half of all dog owners questioned said they had taken their pets on overnight trips in the past year"; some hotels include pet attractions such as a "personalized welcome package for Whiskers," "a veterinarian-approved room-service menu," "homemade biscuits each morning" for dogs, and a "Yappy Hour" for "social critters."[29] A newsletter for people who like to travel with their pet is called "Bone Voyage." People who cannot take their pets along but feel guilty leaving them behind can house them at deluxe pet hotels, now available in many cities. A pet hotel in Washington, D.C., charges $230 per day for a suite "replete with expansive views, 24-hour attendants and tasteful décor accented with original artwork."[30]

Since pets are family members, no expense for their care is considered too great. Americans spend $19 billion on veterinary care, including pet specialists in cardiology, dentistry, ophthalmology, psychotherapy, and radiology. Surgical procedures such as hip replacements and kidney transplants, costing as much as $15,000, have become routine.[31] And if your pet is in danger of dying, you can take some tissue to have it cloned. In 2004, a company called Genetic Savings and Clone announced that it would clone cats for $50,000 each and expected to soon be able to clone dogs as well.[32]

Specialty pet foods and supplies are also big business. Available for purchase are heated dog beds made with designer fabrics, $4,500 dog houses, Irish knit sweaters, jogging suits, National Football League team jerseys, raincoats, fleece boots, and pet pajamas.[33] In Israel, gas masks can be purchased in various sizes for both dogs and cats.[34] Hallmark now markets a death-of-pet card that says, "In sympathy, in your loss of your loving friend," while Internet pet suppliers offer cremation urns, caskets, and memorial stones "to honor your pet until you meet again at the 'Rainbow Bridge.'"[35] When the costs of veterinary care, pet food, and pet supplies are combined, Americans now spend some $47 billion per year on their pets, more than the gross national product of Costa Rica, Guatemala, Ecuador, Ivory Coast, Ethiopia, Croatia, Bulgaria, or Lebanon.[36]

The new relationship between U.S. pet owners and pets is also reflected in the courts. In New York and other cities, there is "a growing group of homeowners and renters who argue that they should be able to keep their pets even if community or building rules forbid them." One New York lawyer "has handled nearly 40 such cases since 2000." In most cases, pet owners argue that their pet is necessary for emotional support. In 2003, the New York City Bar Association began offering a course that "included material on emotional support animals." Also that year, the federal Department of Transportation relaxed rules that prohibited airline passengers from keeping pets with them on airplanes. Pets may now accompany passengers who have letters from their doctors or therapists saying that "the pet is necessary for emotional support."[37]

Viewing pets as integral members of human families is also reflected by legislation introduced in Colorado in 2003 to legally upgrade the status of dogs and cats from "property" to "companions." The purpose, said the sponsors of the legislation, would be to "allow lawsuits against veterinarians or animal abusers for up to $100,000 for loss of companionship and emotional suffering" if a pet is injured or killed.[38] The proposed legislation has not yet been enacted.

The Benefits of Pets

The increasingly close relationship between pets and their owners is partly due to an increasing realization that pets may be beneficial to humans. An obvious example is the use of dogs to assist individuals who are blind or deaf and those with severe physical disabilities such as muscular dystrophy and cerebral palsy. Dogs trained to help the latter, according to a recent survey, can be taught to "open and close doors, turn switches on and off, pull a person up from a sitting or lying down position, assist a person in and out of baths and pools, help pull on clothing, procure and pick up objects, pull wheelchairs, help with shopping, carry parcels, and drag a person to safety in case of fire or other emergency." A study that compared forty-eight disabled individuals who were given service dogs to forty-eight individuals who were not given dogs reported that, at the end of one year, the former had significant improvements in self-esteem, psychological well-being, school attendance, and part-time employment. Equally important, the disabled individuals with service dogs markedly decreased their use of both paid and unpaid human assistants.[39]

There is also increasing evidence that pets can reduce loneliness and depression, especially in individuals who are socially isolated. A survey of 1,992 homosexual and bisexual men reported that "persons with AIDS who owned pets reported less depression than persons with AIDS who did not own pets." The benefit was most significant among individuals who were the most isolated and had the fewest close friends.[40]

Anecdotal data to support such findings are abundant. In New York, a thirty-six-year-old bond salesman claimed that when separated from his black Labrador, he "became a miserable human being in every way that you can think of"; his wife agreed, saying that without the dog, her husband was "depressed and very difficult to live with."[41]

Pets have also been widely used in nursing homes and in institutions for individuals with psychiatric disabilities, where much of their beneficial value has been phrased in terms of companionship: "When older people withdraw from active participation in daily human affairs, the nonhuman environment in general and animals in particular can become increasingly important. Animals have boundless capacity for acceptance, adoration, attention, forgiveness, and unconditional love. Although the potential for significant benefits to a great variety of people exists through association with companion animals, the potential seems greatest in the elderly, for whom the bond with animal companions is perhaps stronger and more profound than at any other age."[42] Studies have shown, for example, that individuals with Alzheimer's disease are less agitated and more social when they have companion animals.[43]

Surveys that ask pet owners why they have pets usually elicit answers that include feelings of security, being loved, being needed, and not being judged. In one study, divorced women who owned dogs said that "whereas husbands may come and go, and children may grow up and leave home, a 'dog is forever'; . . . pets never withhold their love, they never get angry and leave, and they never go out looking for new owners."[44] A study of single women concluded that "a pet can help to diminish feelings of loneliness, particularly for women living alone, and compensate for the absence of human companionship."[45] Similarly, more than half of homeless individuals who kept a pet reported that "relationships with their pets were their only relationships with other human beings." As one writer summarized it: "There is no psychiatrist in the world like a puppy licking your face."[46]

In addition to the psychological benefits of companionship, pets may provide medical benefits. Cat and dog owners, compared to nonowners, have been reported to have lower resting heart rates and blood pressures and to handle conditions of experimental stress better when their pet is present.[47] Two studies of patients with severe cardiac problems reported that the presence of a pet in the home increased the survival rate of such patients. In one of the studies, the benefits were found only when the pet was a dog; a cat provided no beneficial effect.[48] Part of the cardiac benefit in such studies undoubtedly accrues from the necessity of walking the dog, thus affording the owner more exercise.

Companion animals have also been shown to increase the general wellbeing of adults and to decrease their use of physician services. In one study, adults who acquired a new dog or cat, followed for ten months, reported "a highly significant reduction in minor health problems"; the benefit lasted the entire ten-month period for the dog owners but was present only for the first month for cat owners.[49] Similarly, physician use was measured for 938 Medicare enrollees who were undergoing stressful life situations. Those who owned a dog did not see their doctors more often under stressful circumstances, but owning a cat or other pet afforded no such benefit.[50]

It is noteworthy that most studies that report beneficial effects from owning a pet have focused on adults. Few studies have reported benefits of pet ownership for children, except in two major arenas. One is children who have autism, childhood schizophrenia, or other severe psychiatric disabilities; such children have been shown to relate better to companion animals than to adults. For this reason, dogs or other animals are sometime used as "cotherapists" in psychotherapy for such children.[51]

The other major benefit of animal exposure for children is a possible decrease in the likelihood of their getting asthma, hay fever, or other allergies. Some studies have reported that children who are raised on farms have a lower incidence of allergic disorders, but other studies have not replicated these findings. One of the positive studies found that the benefit was greatest when animal exposure started early in life. The benefit was also dose dependent; more exposure produced greater benefit. Thus, small children who were "exposed to stables, farm milk, or both in their first year of life" had the lowest incidence of allergies. "Furthermore, amount and duration of exposure also seemed to play an important part in conferring protection against development of hay fever and allergic sensitization. For asthma, even short exposure times conferred protection."[52] Another study found that exposure to dogs and cats in the first year of life decreased children's chances of later developing asthma or other allergies. Significantly, however, the benefit was seen only if the child was exposed to two or more animals, suggesting that the benefit was not acquired from casual contact alone.[53] Against such possible decrease in allergies with childhood exposure to animals must be weighed the findings that both dogs and cats induce allergies in some children.

Diseases Transmitted by Dogs

Given the increasing number of pet animals and the increasing intimacy between pets and their owners, it is inevitable that an increasing exchange of microbes is also taking place. As noted by William McNeil in *Plagues and People*: "It appears obvious that the sharing of infection increases with the degree of intimacy that prevails between man and beast."[54]

Bites are the most common mode of transmission to humans of microbes from both dogs and cats. "Several million" people in the United States are bitten by dogs and cats each year, "resulting in approximately 300,000 visits to emergency departments, 10,000 hospitalizations, and 20 deaths, mostly among young children."[55] Because cats have such sharp teeth, their bites cause deep puncture wounds and are more likely than dog bites to become infected. A study of infected human wounds from dog and cat bites reported that the median number of different types of bacteria cultured from a single human wound was 5.0 for dogs and 6.5 for cats; however, individual bites from dogs had as many as sixteen different types of bacteria, and from cats, thirteen different types. Most of the bacteria remain localized to the wound, although occasionally they may enter the general circulation and cause serious problems in joints (arthritis), the heart (endocarditis), or the brain (meningitis).[56]

Apart from dog bites, the risk of transmission of serious diseases from dogs to humans appears relatively low. One reason for this is that dogs and humans have had a close relationship for more than ten thousand years, and during that time humans have been exposed to most microbes carried by dogs. It is thus unlikely that there will be many microbial surprises from dogs compared to cats or other pets to which humans have had comparatively less exposure. Diseases known or strongly suspected to be transmissible from dogs to humans are these: bordetellosis, brucellosis, campylobacteriosis, cryptosporidiosis, cutaneous larva migrans, dirofilariasis, echinococcus, giardiasis, leishmaniasis, leptospirosis, Lyme disease (by ticks), rabies, and toxocariasis. Apart from infected dog-bite wounds, the most important dog-associated disease for individuals in the United States is toxocariasis.

The bacterial infection *bordetellosis* is caused by *Bordetella bronchiseptica*, a close cousin of the bacteria that causes pertussis (whooping cough). It is carried by both dogs and cats and is occasionally transmitted to humans, especially children or adults who are immunocompromised. Symptoms include fever, malaise, joint pains, and/or respiratory problems. It can be treated with antibiotics.

Brucellosis is a bacterial disease usually transmitted to humans from cows and other farm animals (see chapter 3). Dogs, however, may also be a reservoir. In humans, it causes fever, malaise, and enlarged lymph nodes. In beagles, it is an important cause of abortions.

The bacterial disease *campylobacteriosis* "has emerged as the most common infectious diarrhea in the United States."[57] It is carried by a variety of wild and domestic animals, with dogs and cats responsible for approximately 6 percent of human cases.[58] The diarrhea may be severe and accompanied by fever. Exposure to dogs or cats with diarrhea increases one's risk of getting this disease. It can be treated with antibiotics.

Responsible for *cryptosporidiosis*, *Cryptosporidium parvum* is a protozoon carried by both dogs and cats and may be transmitted by fecal contamination of food or water. In humans, it causes diarrhea and occurs most commonly in children. Since this parasite is also carried by other animals, the role of dogs and cats in causing this disease is not yet clear. The parasite is a major cause of intestinal disease in individuals who are immunocompromised, such as those with HIV infection.

Cutaneous larva migrans is caused by a type of hookworm carried by dogs and occurs mostly in southern states. Humans may get it by walking barefoot in areas contaminated by dog feces. Once beneath the skin, it causes redness, itching, and swelling of the local area and may slowly spread. It is usually self-limited but may be treated.

Dirofilariasis, caused by the dog heartworm, *Dirofilaria immitis,* is transmitted from dog to dog by mosquitoes, and humans are occasionally accidental hosts. The larvae migrate to the heart and lungs. It is usually asymptomatic, but the worms sometimes form lung nodules that may be mistaken on X-rays for an embolus or lung cancer.

Echinococcus is caused by a tapeworm carried by dogs. When ingested by humans through food or water contaminated with dog feces, the tapeworm may go to the liver or lungs, causing large cysts that may require surgical excision. The disease is rare in the United States, except in southwestern states and Alaska.

Giardiasis is caused by the protozoon *Giardia lamblia,* also a common cause of human diarrhea and usually gotten from contaminated water. It is carried by a variety of animals, including dogs and cats, but rarely causes symptoms in them. Although pet-to-human transmission has not yet been proven, it is strongly suspected.

Dogs, wolves, foxes, and other canids are the natural carriers for protozoa that cause **leishmaniasis**. Leishmaniasis affects five hundred thousand people each year in South America, Asia, and the Middle East. It causes fever with enlarged lymph nodes and is often confused with malaria. A mild skin form of leishmaniasis has infected hundreds of U.S. military personnel in Iraq during the war, where it is widely referred to as the "Baghdad Boil."[59] An especially disfiguring form of the disease, espundia, occurs in South America and causes "the nose and mouth parts [to] literally rot away."[60] Sandflies carry the protozoa from dogs to humans and in some cases from humans to humans; in Italy, Spain, and Brazil, as many as one-quarter of all dogs are infected.[61]

Leishmaniasis is thought to be rare in the United States. However, in 1999, twenty-one foxhounds at a hunt club near New York City died from it, although the outbreak was apparently not transmitted to humans.[62] Subsequent studies have confirmed the occurrence of visceral leishmaniasis in dogs in twenty-one states, thus showing that it is much more widespread than was previously thought and has the potential to cause human disease. In 2000, the Institute of Medicine called visceral leishmaniasis "one of the most important emerging parasitic diseases" and "a major public health problem" because of its increasing incidence in Europe among drug users and immunocompromised individuals with AIDS.[63]

Leptospirosis is caused by a spirochetal bacteria. It may be transmitted to humans by the infected urine of many animals, but most commonly of rats and dogs. It usually occurs in outbreaks when drinking water has been contaminated with the urine of rats or dogs; in 1998, 375 cases of leptospirosis occurred among triathlon participants in the Midwest.[64] Affected individuals may develop a fever, malaise, severe headache, or mild jaundice. In its severe form, it affects the kidneys and liver and is called Weil's disease. It can be treated with antibiotics.

Lyme disease is transmitted from deer to humans by ticks. Occasionally, humans become infected by ticks carried by dogs or cats.

Rabies from infected dogs continues to be a major problem in countries in which rabies vaccine is not routinely given to dogs. In China, for example, rabies from dog bites killed 1,297 people in a nine-month period in 2003, more people than died from SARS or AIDS.[65] In the United States, rabies among dogs and cats is rare; the major carriers of the virus are bats and raccoons, as we will see later in this chapter.

Toxocariasis is "the most common zoonotic infection associated with pet animals in the United States."[66] It is caused by the roundworms *Toxocara canis* from dogs or *Toxocara cati* from cats. The former are more common, and virtually all puppies shed this parasite in their first weeks of life. Deposited in children's outdoor play areas or sandboxes, the parasite eggs remain alive for months and may be ingested by children, especially those who eat dirt. Most infected children show no symptoms but may have a high blood count of eosinophil cells. However, in some cases, the parasite migrates to the lungs or liver, causing cough, wheezing, fever, or an enlarged liver (visceral larva migrans). In other cases, it migrates to the eye (ocular larva migrans) and "causes hundreds of cases of unilateral blindness and less permanent forms of ocular disorders in children each year in the USA."[67] This parasite may also cause some cases of epilepsy, but this has not been proven. Toxocariasis may be prevented by properly disposing of dog and cat feces, keeping unused sandboxes covered, and treating puppies and kittens with deworming medications.

Multiple Sclerosis

Foremost among diseases for which a link between dogs and humans has been suggested but never proven is multiple sclerosis, a chronic disease of the brain that affects approximately 300,000 persons in the United States and 2.5 million worldwide. It begins most commonly between ages twenty and thirty-five, with symptoms such as double vision, clumsiness, weakness of the arms or legs, or changes in sensation. In 10 percent of cases it remains benign for most of the person's life, in 70 percent it relapses and remits as it slowly progresses, and in 20 percent it rapidly progresses to total disability and death.

Infectious agents have been suspected for more than a century to be one of the causes of multiple sclerosis. One reason for this is reports of clusters of cases, which often occur in infectious diseases. Multiple sclerosis also has a striking geographic distribution, with a much higher incidence at latitudes distant from the equator. In addition, there is evidence—based on studies of people who migrate from a country with a high incidence to a country with a low incidence or vice versa—that whatever causes multiple sclerosis gets into the brain before age fifteen and then remains latent for ten years or more. Most important, individuals with multiple sclerosis often have increased antibodies to various viruses and increased immunoglobulins, both of which are measures of infection, in their cerebrospinal fluid. The infectious agent that has been studied most actively is the measles virus; other suspects have included various herpes viruses, rubella, influenza, parainfluenza, and a retrovirus.

One reason animals have been proposed as possible sources of the infectious agent is because multiple sclerosis–like diseases occur in several animal species. As early as 1952, it was suggested that "dogs or cats may be suspected as reservoirs of the [infectious] agent." Animal theories received support in 1977 with a report that three sisters, ages twenty-three to thirty, had all developed multiple sclerosis shortly after their pet dog experienced a severe neurological illness.[68]

This report triggered an outpouring of research studies to ascertain whether individuals with multiple sclerosis had been more exposed to dogs compared to individuals who did not have the disease. One researcher who reported a positive association claimed that this "discovery is of monumental importance, analogous to the discovery of the link between cigarette smoking and cancer." An editorial in a leading neurological journal called 1977 "the year of the dog," and the possible link between multiple sclerosis and dogs was widely reported by the media.[69]

A quarter of a century later, the possible relationship of multiple sclerosis and dogs is still unresolved and continues to stir lively debate among neurologists. At least twenty-one studies have been carried out on dog exposure. In seven of them, individuals with multiple sclerosis had significantly more exposure to dogs than the controls; in the remaining studies, no significant association was found, but in none of them did the controls have significantly more dog exposure. In some studies, only small dogs or dogs kept in the house appeared to be risk factors.[70]

Several of the studies inquired specifically about exposure to sick dogs before the onset of human multiple sclerosis. This is of special interest because dogs may be infected with the canine distemper virus, which is closely related to the human measles virus. Some researchers have claimed that epidemics of canine distemper in dogs have been followed by outbreaks of multiple sclerosis in humans, including outbreaks in the Faroe Islands; Iceland;

Newfoundland; Key West, Florida; and Sitka, Alaska.[71] In Sitka, for example, an outbreak of distemper occurred among dogs in 1965. Between 1967 and 1970, five individuals with a multiple sclerosis–like illness were diagnosed, the only such cases diagnosed in Sitka between 1949 and 1979.[72] Based on such observations, several research groups have tested individuals with multiple sclerosis to see whether they have increased antibodies to the canine distemper virus. A 1997 summary of such studies concluded that "the evidence for an etiologic role for canine distemper virus in MS [multiple sclerosis] is at best equivocal."[73]

Such studies have many methodological problems, and the results remain controversial. Dogs are so widely distributed as pets that almost everyone has owned or been exposed to them at the homes of relatives and neighbors. The issue of timing of exposure also continues to be problematic; since there is probably a latent period of several years between exposure to the dog and disease onset, one must measure dog exposure at various times in the past and follow humans for an extended period of time to ascertain whether they develop the disease.

Diseases Transmitted by Cats

Since cats have been widely used as pets for less than two hundred years, human exposure to feline microbes has occurred for a relatively short period. Diseases transmitted from cats to humans are these: bordetellosis, campylobacteriosis, cat scratch disease, cryptosporidiosis, giardiasis, Lyme disease (by ticks), plague (by fleas), rabies, toxocariasis, and toxoplasmosis. Except for infected cat-bite wounds, discussed earlier, the most important cat-associated diseases for individuals in the United States are cat-scratch disease, toxocariasis, and especially toxoplasmosis. (Discussion of several of the diseases listed can be found in the section on dog-associated diseases.)

There are approximately twenty-two thousand cases of cat-scratch disease, including two thousand hospitalizations, each year in the United States.[74] The cause of cat-scratch disease eluded investigators for many years. However, recent studies show that it is caused by a bacteria, *Bartonella henselae*, transmitted to humans by the scratch or bite of a cat or, occasionally, by cat fleas. It usually affects children and is most commonly acquired from young or stray cats. A sore (papule) at the site of inoculation is followed by enlarged lymph nodes and mild fever. Most cases are self-limited, but a few progress to involve other organs, including the heart, lungs, liver, eyes, and brain. It can be treated with antibiotics, although the response to the medication varies.

Plague is a bacterial disease (*Yersina pestis*) that in the United States mostly occurs among rodents in southwestern states (see chapter 6). Cats may become infected by contact with infected rodents. In New Mexico between 1977 and 1988, 119 cases of plague in cats were reported. Cats occasionally transmit it to humans, usually by carrying plague-infected fleas. Of the 297 cases of human plague in the United States between 1977 and 1998, 23 were believed to have been transmitted by cats; in 5 of those cases, the outcome was fatal because of a failure to properly diagnose the person and begin antibiotics.[75]

Toxoplasmosis is caused by a protozoa, *Toxoplasma gondii*, which over millions of years has adapted to cats and other felids. Cats rarely show symptoms, but when first infected they may pass up to twenty million cysts per day in their feces. The cysts are extremely hardy and may remain infective in soil or sand for up to eighteen months. If the cysts are ingested by other animals, they may go to muscle tissue and remain there. If that animal is in turn eaten by a felid, the cysts complete their complex life cycle in the cat. A special situation occurs when *Toxoplasma* is ingested by a mammal that is pregnant. In such situations, the microbe may infect the placenta or cross the placenta and infect the fetus. This is a major cause of spontaneous abortions among sheep and may also cause severe problems for the human fetus.

Humans become infected with *Toxoplasma gondii* by inhalation or ingestion. Inhalation of cysts may occur in anyone who is exposed to cat feces, such as when they are deposited in litter boxes, under chairs, in gardens, in loose soil around the house, or in children's sandboxes. The feces become dry within two days, lose their color and odor within two weeks, and can no longer be distinguished from the surrounding soil or sand. Cysts from infected cats may become airborne and thus inhaled when the dried feces are disturbed, as when a person changes the cat litter, digs in the garden, or plays in the sandbox.

Sandboxes (called "sandpits" in many countries) should be regarded as common sources of *Toxoplasma* infection for children, since studies have shown many of them to be highly contaminated with cat feces. In one study of three public sandboxes in urban parks, a total of 176 cat defecations took place over a four-week period, mostly at night.[76] Since a single infected cat can deposit millions of cysts per day, and since the cysts can remain infective in moist sand or soil for as long as eighteen months, it seems likely that many children playing in such sandboxes become infected.

A second major route by which humans may become infected with *Toxoplasma* is by eating undercooked meat from animals that became infected by ingesting cysts from cat feces. The muscles of these infected animals contain microscopic cysts that can be transmitted to humans or other animals if the muscle is eaten. This is a common mode of infection in countries such as France, Germany, Turkey, Pakistan, Sudan, and Ethiopia, where undercooked meat is widely consumed. The effectiveness of transmitting *Toxoplasma* by undercooked meat was demonstrated in a study of a children's institution in France: Given "barely cooked beef or horse meat" and "undercooked lamb chops," 100 percent of the children demonstrated antibodies to *Toxoplasma* at the end of one year.[77]

Humans may also become infected with *Toxoplasma* by drinking contaminated water or milk or by ingesting unwashed fruits or vegetables that have been exposed to flies or cockroaches carrying *Toxoplasma* cysts. Houseflies have been shown to infect food with *Toxoplasma* for up to two days after the flies have had contact with infected cat feces. Cockroaches may excrete *Toxoplasma* in their feces for up to ten days after ingesting infected cat feces.[78]

What are the chances of humans becoming infected with *Toxoplasma* from these various sources? In the United States, studies have shown that approximately 1 percent of cats are actively infected, and thus shedding cysts, at any one time. Studies of how many cats have ever been infected, as measured by the presence of antibodies against *Toxoplasma*, have shown the number to be approximately one-third.[79] The infection rate is lower in cats kept indoors and higher in stray cats, since the latter rely more on hunting for their food and thus are more likely to ingest infected rodents. Cats excrete cysts only at the time they acquire their initial infection. In young cats, this is most likely to take place when they become old enough to begin hunting for themselves; thus, excretion of cysts is much more likely to occur in cats at this stage of development. A study of pregnant women in Norway attempted to assess the relative importance of various factors for becoming infected with *Toxoplasma*. It reported that the women who became infected had a significantly greater exposure to cat litter boxes, undercooked meats, and raw fruits and vegetables; thus, multiple sources of infection appear to be important.[80]

The number of humans who have been infected by *Toxoplasma gondii*, as measured by their having antibodies, varies geographically depending on cat exposure and dietary habits. A national survey in the United States reported that 23 percent of people are infected.[81] By contrast, a survey of pregnant women in Paris, where undercooked meat is highly valued, reported that 84 percent of them had been infected.[82] High rates have also been reported in countries where cats are numerous and exposure to their feces is thought to be common.[83]

Clinically, the best-studied form of human toxoplasmosis is the congenital form, which occurs when *Toxoplasma* infects a pregnant woman who has not previously been infected. In the United States, "approximately one out of every 1,000 pregnant women becomes infected, resulting in anywhere from 400 to 4,000 cases of congenital toxoplasmosis each year."[84] In approximately 60 percent of such cases, the parasite infects the mother but causes no symptoms and does not affect the placenta or fetus. In the other 40 percent, *Toxoplasma* affects the placenta and fetus, causing spontaneous abortion or stillbirth in approximately 5 percent of cases and congenital toxoplasmosis at birth in an additional 10 percent. The symptoms of congenital toxoplasmosis may include changes in head size (hydrocephaly or microcephaly), cysts in the brain, mental retardation, deafness, seizures, cerebral palsy, enlargement of the liver and spleen, and damage to the retina.

The remaining 25 percent of children infected with *Toxoplasma* in utero appear normal at birth but develop symptoms later. In most cases, this form of toxoplasmosis involves infections of the eyes (retina and choroid), which may produce scarring or impaired vision. Symptoms in these delayed-onset cases peak in the person's second and third decade of life. Much of the damage in congenitally transmitted toxoplasmosis can be prevented by timely treatment with appropriate antibiotics if the correct diagnosis is made.

Acquired toxoplasmosis occurs when *Toxoplasma* infects a nonpregnant person for the first time, most commonly a child or young adult. It may cause no symptoms or manifest as headache, fever, and enlarged lymph nodes, symptoms often misdiagnosed as a cold, flu, mononucleosis, or other disorder. In some cases, acquired toxoplasmosis may proceed to a relapsing or chronic stage and cause more serious symptoms. Such symptoms may include infection of the liver (hepatitis), heart muscle (myocarditis), brain (encephalitis), lungs (pneumonia), or eye (retinochoroiditis). In one study of seventy cases of acquired toxoplasmosis, these more serious symptoms occurred in twenty-six patients.[85]

In addition to the congenital and acquired forms of toxoplasmosis, a third form occurs in individuals with an impaired immune system, including those receiving chemotherapy for cancer and those infected with HIV. Infection of the brain with toxoplasmosis occurs in approximately 30 percent of AIDS patients who have had a previous primary infection and causes up to 10 percent of deaths in these patients.[86] The cerebral toxoplasmosis may cause eye disease and a variety of neurological and psychiatric symptoms, including seizures, cranial nerve palsies, focal neurological signs, and altered mental status such as confusion, delusions, and hallucinations.[87] The toxoplasmosis in such immunocompromised individuals is a reactivation of latent *Toxoplasma* that has lain dormant in the body, often for many years.

The activation of latent toxoplasmosis in individuals with AIDS has led to a realization that "*Toxoplasma gondii* is among the most prevalent causes of latent infection of the central nervous system (CNS) throughout the world" and has raised questions about what else it might be doing in human brains.[88] In sheep, pigs, and cattle, *Toxoplasma* causes neurological symptoms. Studies of mice and rats have shown that infection with *Toxoplasma* decreases their memory and learning ability.[89] Of special interest are the studies of Joanne Webster and her colleagues in England, which show that *Toxoplasma*-infected rats become more active and lose their natural aversion to the smell of cats, behaviors that increase the chances that such rats will be eaten by cats. Since this would return the *Toxoplasma gondii* cyst to cats, where it can effectively complete its life cycle, this altered behavior has been used as an example of evolutionarily derived manipulation by the parasite.[90]

In humans, *Toxoplasma* may cause mental retardation, and there has been speculation that it may also cause some cases of epilepsy, Guillain-Barré syndrome, and brain tumors such as meningiomas.[91] Also of interest are studies suggesting that toxoplasmosis infections in otherwise normal individuals may produce subtle changes in personality traits, impairment in psychomotor skills, and a lowering of IQ.[92]

Recent research has also focused on the possibility that *Toxoplasma gondii* may play a role in the causation of severe psychiatric disorders. Such research was stimulated by observations that AIDS patients who have reactivated toxoplasmosis have delusions, hallucinations, and other manifestations of disordered thought processes. There are also reports of such psychiatric symptoms in individuals with acquired toxoplasmosis; in a review of 114 such cases, "psychiatric disturbances were very frequent" in 24 of them.[93]

Nineteen studies have been carried out that assess antibodies to *Toxoplasma gondii* in individuals with schizophrenia and other severe psychiatric disorders; all except one of the studies reported that patients had more antibodies than control groups had.[94] A study of mothers who gave birth to individuals who later developed schizophrenia and other psychoses reported that the mothers, in blood taken just prior to delivery, had more antibodies to *Toxoplasma* than mothers whose offspring did not develop these disorders.[95] Finally, two studies have ascertained that individuals with a diagnosis of schizophrenia or bipolar disorder were more likely to have owned a cat during childhood than individuals without such diagnoses.[96] Studies relating *Toxoplasma* infection to severe psychiatric disorders are ongoing, including studies to assess whether treatment for *Toxoplasma* results in clinically apparent improvement for some individuals with these diseases.

Another human disease for which there has been speculation regarding the possible role of cats is rheumatoid arthritis. This is a disease of joints, affecting women more often than men and usually becoming manifest after the age of forty. It is widely accepted that some individuals have a genetic predisposition to rheumatoid arthritis and that there are abnormalities in such persons' immune systems. Some researchers have also suspected that an infectious agent triggers the disease, and a variety of microbes has been proposed.

If rheumatoid arthritis is triggered by an infectious agent, could the agent be transmitted from animals? The first group to ask that question was Norman Gottlieb and his colleagues at the University of Miami. In a 1974 study, they compared pet histories for the five years preceding the onset of illness for 105 individuals with rheumatoid arthritis, 105 individuals with other forms of arthritis, and 95 individuals with nonarthritic illnesses. They found that "the rheumatoid group had significantly greater exposure to one or more dogs, cats, or birds (combined) than did the arthritic controls." When the pets were analyzed individually, the presence of a pet dog or any sick animal in the home of an individual with rheumatoid arthritis was statistically significant. There were also "more cats and birds in the homes of patients who developed RA [rheumatoid arthritis], but differences were not statistically significant."[97]

In 1996, Colin Bond and Leslie Cleland at the University of Adelaide, Australia, followed up the Gottlieb study. They compared the animal exposure histories for 122 individuals with rheumatoid arthritis and 114 individuals with other arthritides, mostly osteoarthritis. They asked about a broad array of animals, including dogs, cats, rabbits, guinea pigs, mice, parakeets, cockatoos, parrots, pigeons, fish, ducks, sheep, cattle, pigs, goats, and horses. Their most significant finding was that individuals with rheumatoid arthritis had a statistically significant greater exposure to cats, especially in the five years before puberty. Exposure to parakeets also achieved significance, but exposure to none of the other animals was significantly different between the two groups.[98] No additional studies on animal exposure in rheumatoid arthritis have been reported since this study.

Other Pets

Although dogs and cats are the most popular choices as pets, fish, rabbits, birds, and small rodents are also widely kept.

Aquarium fish can be found in more than twenty million homes in the United States. They are considered to be "relatively harmless" in terms of human disease risk.[99] The most common disease transmitted by fish is a skin infection caused by mycobacteria, and it occurs most often when persons cleaning the fish tank have cuts on their hands.

Rabbits, when raised domestically rather than caught in the wild, are also considered "exceptionally free of most transmittable zoonoses" and can be trained to make good pets.[100] If improperly restrained, rabbits will sometimes inflict painful scratches with their back feet, and the scratches may become infected. Wild rabbits, however, should not be kept as pets, since they may carry tularemia (see chapter 3). Approximately one hundred cases of human tularemia occur in the United States each year from wild rabbits. Especially ironic was a case in which a father gave the rabbit feet from a wild rabbit to his two children as good luck charms; both children developed tularemia.[101]

Caged birds are commonly kept as pets but present some risks to their owners. Allergic reactions, including asthma attacks, are relatively common in owners. Caged birds may also spread salmonellosis, giardiasis, influenza (see chapter 9), and Newcastle disease, an influenza-like syndrome caused by a paramyxovirus. One of the most serious diseases they may transmit is psittacosis.

Psittacosis, also known as parrot fever, is caused by a bacteria, *Chlamydia psittaci*, and may be carried by almost all bird species, including parrots, parakeets, cockatiels, canaries, and finches. A study of pet birds in Florida found that 20 percent of them were infected.[102]

Psittacosis is often asymptomatic in birds, and it is believed that some birds carry the bacteria throughout their lifetime. Situations that cause stress, such as crowding birds in cages and transporting them, may cause latent bacteria to become active and cause symptomatic disease. The symptoms of psittacosis in birds vary by species, as well as by strain of bacteria, but include inflammation of the eyes, nasal discharge, diarrhea, lethargy, and ruffled feathers. Some infected birds may die, especially if they are subjected to stress; others recover but have periodic relapses; and others recover completely.

Chlamydia psittaci is transmitted from birds to humans most commonly when humans inhale droplets of dried bird excreta that have become airborne. Birds excrete bacteria in their eyes, nasal secretions, and feces and may carry it on their feathers. Studies have shown that one may become infected merely by being in the same room with an infected bird, and infections have been reported among multiple family members infected from a single bird, as well as among individuals visiting a bird park.[103] "Kissing or nuzzling the bird, handling the bird, and feeding the bird" have been shown to increase the chances of transmission.[104] Intimate exposure to pet birds markedly increases transmission, as demonstrated by the odd case of "a man who developed life-threatening psittacosis after administering 'mouth to beak' resuscitation to his ill, newly purchased parrot."[105] There are suggestions that *Chlamydia psittaci* may occasionally be transmitted from person to person, although this has not been proven.[106]

Human psittacosis is varied in its manifestations, from being asymptomatic to being a fatal disease.[107] Classically, the infected person develops influenza-like symptoms of chills, fever, headache, muscle aches, and malaise. This may be followed by coughing, chest pain, shortness of breath, and pneumonia. The pneumonia caused by *Chlamydia psittaci* may be severe;[108] it may also look similar to pneumonia caused by another member of the Chlamydia family, *Chlamydia pneumonia*. Occasionally, *Chlamydia psittaci* also infects other organs, including the heart, liver, kidney, joints, and brain. Before the availability of antibiotics, the mortality rate from human *Chlamydia psittaci* infections was over 20 percent, but it is now less than 1 percent.[109]

The most worrisome aspect of *Chlamydia psittaci*, however, is what other human diseases it may be setting off. In the animal kingdom, it has been implicated in causing pneumonia, arthritis, diarrhea and inflammation of the intestine, and abortions.[110] In humans, *Chlamydia psittaci* may be responsible for some cases of temporal arteritis and temperomandibular joint syndrome, but this has not yet been established and the cases may represent cross-reactions to another closely related *Chlamydia*.[111] As is true for other members of the Chlamydia family, there is a general belief among researchers that we are just beginning to understand how many human diseases these bacteria may cause.

Small rodents raised domestically, such as hamsters, gerbils, guinea pigs, mice, and rats, can also make good pets. Since they have been used in laboratory research for many years, we know a great deal about diseases they may carry. They are not without risk, however, and may induce allergies in some people. They may also carry a variety of infectious agents, although those causing the most serious diseases, such as plague, typhus, and hantavirus infection, occur in wild rodents but not generally in rodents raised for sale.

One important microbe that pet rodents may carry is the virus that causes lymphocytic choriomeningitis (LCM). LCM virus is a member of the arenavirus family, which also contains the lethal Lassa fever virus and several viruses that cause viral hemorrhagic fevers. Hamsters and mice do not show any signs of illness following infection with the LCM virus, suggesting that these species have carried the virus for a long period of time. They may transmit the virus to a human who handles the animal or is simply around its cage, since the virus, shed in the rodent's urine and feces, may become airborne.

In most cases, LCM causes a relatively mild illness, with fever, headache, muscle aches, eye pain, and nausea and vomiting. However, in approximately one-third of human cases, LCM also causes meningitis or encephalitis, with severe headache, stiff neck, and other neurological symptoms. LCM infections are rarely fatal but occur in humans more frequently than was previously thought. One study of a rural population in northern Germany, where mice are relatively common, reported that 9 percent of the population had been exposed to LCM, as measured by their having antibodies against it.[112]

Pet hamsters have caused outbreaks of human LCM. In one outbreak in New York State, fifty-seven cases of LCM meningitis occurred in a four-month period, with the victims ranging in age from three to seventy. The highest infection rates occurred in households in which hamsters were kept in open wire cages in living rooms or other common living areas.[113] Family outbreaks have also been described, including one in which the husband developed meningitis; his mother-in-law, encephalitis; and his wife and daughter, lesser degrees of illness—all four had handled the family's pet hamster.[114] A hospital outbreak of LCM infection occurred among personnel who visited a room that housed a copy machine and cages of hamsters being used for research. Another outbreak occurred among personnel in a research laboratory using hamsters; two of the seven affected individuals required hospitalization.[115]

LCM infections in humans may be more serious, at least occasionally. When the illness infects pregnant women, it may cross the placenta and has been documented to cause miscarriages and death of the newborn.[116] LCM virus is also known to cause lymphomas in animals and to increase animals' susceptibility to tumors.[117]

Increasing Exposure to Pets and Farm Animals

In addition to an increasing number of pet animals in the United States, there also appears to be an increasing number of feral animals, especially cats. These animals were originally obtained as pets but later ran away or were abandoned. Most feral cats live in wooded areas or vacant buildings. There are also estimated to be approximately two million feral pigs in the United States, predominantly in Texas and other southern states.[118]

The number of feral cats in the United States may be as high as sixty million but is really unknown.[119] As one observer noted, "Counting cats is only slightly less difficult than herding them."[120] In general, however, most estimates of the number of cats in the United States—pet and feral—are at least one hundred million, or one cat for every three persons. Feral animals pose special problems in the transmission of animal microbes, because they "come in contact with both domestic animals and wildlife [and] they can act as conduits for pathogen exchange between otherwise isolated host populations."[121]

It is not necessary, however, to own pet animals to be exposed to them. Children in the United States are exposed to animals at petting farms and petting zoos, which have become increasingly popular in recent years. A Web site devoted to them describes the merits of taking children to places such as Old MacDonald's Petting Zoo, Happy Times Farm, and Country Critters Petting Zoo, which claims to have the "cutest critters in town." Most petting zoos include goats, sheep, rabbits, ducks, pigs, calves, donkeys, ponies, and other farm animals, but some also include more exotic animals. For example, WOW Animals in Sunland, California, advertises "50 species of mammals, birds, reptiles, amphibians and invertebrates."[122]

In many areas, a petting farm or a petting zoo will come to you. Mobile Menagerie in Gilbert, Arizona, suggests that you "reserve a bunch of cute critters for your party or event." Zoo-to-You in Leesburg, Virginia, will bring a "baby zoo" (ducks, chicks, bunnies, and a goat or lamb) or a "full zoo" (plus sheep, donkeys, and llamas) to your child's birthday party for only $200 (baby zoo) or $550 (full zoo) plus a mileage fee.[123] Other events advertised as appropriate for inclusion of a petting zoo are company picnics, church festivals, and school fairs or carnivals. In what was probably a first, the University of Louisiana at Lafayette in 2002 put a petting zoo in the parking lot of its football stadium to increase attendance at one of its home games. According to a news report: "That game drew 20,512 fans, about a third more than their average attendance of 15,056."[124]

The number of children exposed to animals at petting farms or petting zoos is impressive. A popular petting farm near Philadelphia, Pennsylvania, for example, claimed to attract 1,500 to 2,000 persons each day. Most visitors are young children, and most of them have direct contact with the animals by petting or holding them, often to have their picture taken. This petting farm came under scrutiny by public health authorities in late 2000, when fifty-one cases of severe diarrhea occurred among its visitors. All except four of those who became sick were ten years old or younger. Among them, sixteen had to be hospitalized and eight developed kidney failure with a hemolytic uremic syndrome; of these, one child required a kidney transplant. The cause of the outbreak was found to be the 0157 strain of *Escherichia coli* bacteria (see chapter 8), which was carried by cows at the farm. Children who became sick had spent more time with the animals, were less likely to have washed their hands after doing so, and were more likely to have purchased and eaten food from the petting farm's concession stand.[125]

There are no general data available on how frequently children become ill after visits to petting farms or petting zoos. The Pennsylvania outbreak, however, was not unique. Similar outbreaks caused by the same strain of bacteria have been reported in Washington, Wisconsin, England, and Canada; the Canadian outbreak involved 159 visitors.[126] On May 6, 2002, *Inside Edition* aired a program that featured outbreaks of illness at petting zoos. As part of the story, the producers visited eight petting zoos in Florida; none of the eight informed visitors that they might get sick from the animals, but three of the petting zoos had signs warning that the animals could get sick from the visitors.[127]

Exotic Pets

Throughout history and in many cultures, individuals have kept exotic animals as pets. Some ancient Egyptians attempted to tame gazelles, hartebeests, and hyenas, and Moghul emperors in India kept cheetahs as pets. Australian aborigines tamed wallabies, and North American Indians occasionally kept pet bears. Indeed, even a president of the United States, John Quincy Adams, is alleged to have "kept a pet alligator in the East Room bathtub" of the White House.[128]

What is new is not the keeping of exotic pets but rather its rapidly increasing incidence. One estimate is that the sale of exotic pets in the United States is now a billion-dollar-a-year industry.[129] The combination of animals available on the Internet and overnight delivery service has made almost any animal available to any person. Purchasing exotic animals may be seen as an effective way to assert one's individuality, as the National Alternative Pet Association also implies on its Web site: "Is your pet unconventional? Do people put you down because your pet isn't a socially acceptable cat, dog or goldfish? . . . Let's help people understand and love our misunderstood alternative pets."[130]

Ferrets are a good example of an exotic pet that has risen rapidly in popularity. They have been used for hundreds of years as rat hunters, leading to use of the term "to ferret something out." In the United States, there are an estimated "5 to 7 million pet ferrets in approximately 4 to 5 million households nationwide."[131] A Web site, www.ferretstore.com, sells clothing for pet ferrets, including lace hats, raincoats, sweaters, T-shirts, tuxedo shirts, and Santa Claus suits. Ferrets, however, have been known to severely injure small children and can be infected with influenza, rabies, tuberculosis, leptospirosis, listeriosis, salmonellosis, campylobacteriosis, and cryptosproidiosis, although only influenza has been proven so far to have been transmitted to humans.[132]

Ferrets have become so commonplace that many people no longer consider them exotic. To own a *truly* exotic pet these days, one must purchase an animal such as an African pouch rat, bushbaby, bushy-tailed jird, capybara, coatimundi, degus, desert jerboa, fennec fox, fire-bellied toad, gundi, hedgehog, kinkajou, miniature Sicilian donkey, porcupine, serval, sloth, or wallaby. All of these and many others are available for purchase through exotic pet Web sites. If money and space are not limiting factors, one may choose to own large exotic animals. In October 2003, New York City police removed a 425-pound Bengal tiger and an alligator from an apartment in Harlem.[133] Also available for sale on the Internet are buffalo ($2,000), chimpanzees ($55,000), giraffes ($60,000), jaguars ($5,000), kangaroos ($6,000), reindeer ($2,700), and spotted leopards ($3,900).[134] Since it is difficult to imagine a buffalo or reindeer as a companion animal, it seems reasonable to assume that individuals who purchase such animals do so to satisfy other needs.

The recent increase in keeping exotic animals as pets has occurred not only in the United States but also in Europe, Asia, South America, and Africa. The international aspect of this phenomenon is illustrated by a news account of a German family that for thirty-three years kept a pet eel in the bathtub.

"'He's part of our family,' said Hannelore Richter of Bochum, whose husband caught the eel on a fishing trip in 1969 and took it home for supper." However, plans changed when "their children fell in love with it." The family said they had "trained it to swim into a bucket when somebody needs to bathe."[135]

What most exotic pet Web sites and pet stores do not advertise, however, is that exotic pets come with exotic and not-so-exotic diseases. All exotic animals should be regarded as high-risk pets because of their potential for transmitting disease-causing microbes to their human owners. Iguanas, raccoons, and prairie dogs are exotic pets that illustrate this problem.

Pet iguanas are part of what has been called "an explosion of pet reptile ownership in the United States."[136] Lizards, snakes, turtles, and alligators have also increased in popularity. Between 1991 and 2001, the number of U.S. households with reptiles doubled to 1.7 million.[137] A federal inspector reported in 2004 that he was seeing shipments of monitor lizards arriving "almost weekly" and that "it was not uncommon to get shipments of 1,000 baby boas from Colombia or pythons from Indonesia."[138] One 2003 news account, for example, described a Connecticut couple, the Boykos, who kept three five-foot-long alligators in their home as pets. When authorities tried to confiscate the alligators, Mr. Boyko protested. "We didn't have kids," he explained. "We had gators."[139]

Iguanas are found in Central and South America and raised for export on farms in Colombia and El Salvador. U.S. imports of iguanas increased thirtyfold between 1986 and 1993 to almost eight hundred thousand per year.[140] Like all reptiles, iguanas have been infected with salmonella bacteria for millions of years and are asymptomatic carriers of this microbe. As we will see, infection with salmonella usually causes diarrhea, nausea, vomiting, and abdominal cramping, although in small children and individuals who have compromised immune systems the illness can be much more severe. A 1993 study of reptile-associated salmonella infections in New York State found approximately seven hundred cases; in 83 percent of cases the reptile was an iguana.[141] If these figures are representative of the United States as a whole, there were approximately sixteen thousand iguana-associated cases of human salmonella infection that year.

The most serious cases of iguana-associated salmonella infections in the United States have been reported in very young children. For example, in Wisconsin in 1998, a five-month-old boy died suddenly at home from septicemia due to *Salmonella marina*; a family pet iguana was found to be infected with the same microbe.[142] Salmonella-related deaths attributed to iguanas were also reported for a three-week-old infant in Indiana and a newborn baby in New York.[143] The importance of a compromised immune system was illustrated in Massachusetts in 1997, when "an 8-year-old boy with a congenital immune deficiency developed severe vomiting, abdominal cramps, bloody diarrhea and headache" attributed to salmonella infection from two iguanas purchased three days before the onset of the boy's illness.[144] Adults are less likely to develop severe forms of salmonellosis from reptiles but may do so; in Connecticut in 1995, for example, a forty-year-old man developed osteomyelitis, a chronic bone infection, from a salmonella infection he acquired from the family's iguanas.[145]

In reviewing such cases, the manner of transmission of salmonella from iguanas to family members is a cause for concern. In most instances, the young children had no direct contact with the iguanas; rather, the infection was transmitted to them by family members. In some cases, it was established that "the infant's mother fed the iguana and cleaned its cage" and "reported handwashing after these activities."[146] In one case, the infant's father and pet iguana did not even live with the boy, "but his father reported pacifying his son by allowing him to suck his fingers during visits to the child's house."[147] Other children have become infected at the homes of babysitters who owned iguanas or at a birthday party at a home in which iguanas were kept.[148]

Raccoons have attractive masklike faces and ringed tails and are sold on Internet pet sites as exotic pets. They are also the major reservoir for rabies in the United States. In the Middle Atlantic and New England states, rabies is epidemic among them.

Rabies is caused by a virus spread by exposure to the saliva or bite of an infected animal. Once infected, a person experiences muscle spasms, confusion, hallucinations, coma, and death in almost every case. This inevitable course can be reversed only by treating the infected person with rabies vaccine and prophylactic immune globulin after the exposure occurs but before symptoms begin. In the United States, such rabies prophylaxis is given approximately forty thousand times each year at an annual cost of $60 million.[149]

The present epidemic of raccoon rabies in the northeastern United States began in 1977 when, according to one account, "several members of [President] Carter's cabinet and personal staff missed going 'coon hunting' over the weekend, [so] they had some raccoons imported into Virginia from Georgia."[150] More than 3,500 raccoons were translocated for hunting, some of which had rabies.[151] In 1977, raccoons accounted for just 2 percent of all rabid animals in the Middle Atlantic states, but by 1983 they accounted for 84 percent.[152] Dogs and cats, by contrast, accounted for less than 2 percent. Bats, skunks, foxes, coyotes, woodchucks, and beavers may also become infected with rabies; a reportedly rabid beaver "exhibited aggressive behavior by charging canoes and kayaks" on a river.[153]

As the epidemic of raccoon rabies has spread in northeastern states, there has also occurred an inevitable increase in the number of individuals exposed to sick raccoons; these individuals must therefore undergo injections of rabies vaccine and prophylactic immune globulin. In one case, "a baby raccoon was passed between two families and handled by many neighborhood children, exposing 16 persons." In another, "a science teacher encouraged a student to bring his pet raccoon to school." In Florida, a pet raccoon "accounted for the prophylaxis of 172 persons at a cost of more than $64,000."[154] In New Hampshire, a cat infected by a rabid raccoon exposed 665 people, and in New York a goat infected by a rabid raccoon exposed 438 people.[155]

In February 2003, the first human case of rabies from a raccoon was reported. A twenty-five-year-old man in northern Virginia died after two weeks of hospitalization. Molecular studies established that the rabies virus had come from a raccoon, despite the man's having had no known exposure to pet or wild raccoons.[156] It is still not known how he became infected. While attempts are made to bring rabies under control by animal immunization, the increased popularity of pet raccoons has led to new health hazards to humans.

Prairie dogs, foot-long rodents related to squirrels and marmots, became popular as exotic pets in the 1990s. Although no figures are available on the total number of pet prairie dogs in the United States, "officials estimate that 20,000 prairie dogs a year are exported from Texas alone to be sold as pets."[157] They also became popular as pets in Japan until they were banned from that country because they carry not only monkeypox, but also tularemia and plague.[158]

In June 2003, an outbreak of monkeypox occurred in Midwestern states among individuals who had had contact with pet prairie dogs. Symptoms of monkeypox include a high fever, cough, enlarged lymph nodes, and a rash that looks like smallpox. This is not surprising, since the virus that causes monkeypox is in the orthopoxvirus family and closely related to the virus that causes smallpox. Monkeypox outbreaks in Africa have had mortality rates of up to 10 percent. In the U.S. outbreak, one-quarter of the eighty-six cases required hospitalization, but there were no deaths.

Since monkeypox had never been reported anywhere except in Africa before June 2003, an immediate investigation was undertaken by health authorities to ascertain its origin. They discovered that the infected prairie dogs had come from an animal distributor in Illinois who had housed prairie dogs in close proximity to Gambian pouch rats and other rodents imported from Africa; several of these rodents were found to be carriers of the monkeypox virus.

Gambian pouch rats, which are the size of small cats, have hamsterlike pouches and have also become popular in the United States as exotic pets. An Internet Web site describes them as "very intelligent, . . . [with] the ability to bond/show deep affection to their human companions. . . . When the pouches are full it gives the pouch rat an absolutely adorable, yet comical face. If you like rodents, especially rats, they are sure to captivate your heart."[159] No information is available on the number of Gambian pouch rats imported into the United States each year, but the shipment from Africa that included the infected rats consisted of "about 800 small mammals of nine different species, including . . . rope squirrels, tree squirrels, Gambian pouch rats, brushtail porcupines, dormice, and striped mice."[160]

It is not yet known whether the 2003 U.S. monkeypox outbreak was fully contained. Squirrels, not monkeys, are the natural reservoir of the virus in Africa; the disease acquired its name because it often kills monkeys. It is known that in the U.S. outbreak, monkeypox spread to a pet rabbit in one of the homes. Attempts to trace all of the possibly infected prairie dogs proved difficult because, in addition to having been sold in pet stores, they were exchanged at pet "swap meets," at which no sales records are kept.

Public health officials are concerned about the possible spread of monkeypox to pet hamsters, gerbils, or other pet rodents. Even worse, if an infected pet prairie dog had been released in the wild, it could have transmitted the disease to squirrels, chipmunks, rats, and wild prairie dogs, which would permanently establish the disease among U.S. wildlife, similar to what occurred with the plague bacteria a century earlier.

The 2003 U.S. monkeypox outbreak did have one beneficial effect: It focused public attention on the widespread and largely unregulated sale of exotic animals as pets. Several states subsequently banned the sale of prairie dogs, and the federal government restricted the importation of some African rodents. Perhaps the definitive word on the prairie-dog outbreak appeared in an editorial in the June 11, 2003, *New York Times:* "Domestic life is not appropriate for any creature of the wild, whether it is a lion cub or a Gambian rat. And prairie dogs are appropriate pets only for people who own a prairie."

8

C H A P T E R

Humans as Diners

Mad Cows and Sane Chickens

> *Man occupies a unique position in the pecking order of nature. Not only is he able to use anything that he wants as a source of food, but under ordinary circumstances he need not fall prey to any living creature of another species. . . . There is only one significant exception to his biological dominance, but a very large one. Like any other living thing, man can become the victim of microorganisms, and in fact these account for a large percentage of his diseases.*
>
> RENE DUBOS, *Mirage of Health*

HUMANS have been infected with animal microbes since we first began to eat animal meat in the Paleolithic period. Paleolithic man acquired many animal macroparasites, such as taenia and trichinosis, as well as bacteria that cause such diseases as brucellosis, tularemia, and glanders. Humans have thus been exposed to animal microbes over thousands of years by eating animals' meat and drinking their milk, and through animal fecal contamination of food and water. In biblical times, many of the Mosaic laws that governed food consumption and animal care, as detailed in Deuteronomy and Leviticus, were attempts to limit the spread of food-borne and other diseases from animals to humans.

Until recently, human exposure to animal microbes through meat, milk, or contamination was a local affair. Cattle and chickens were raised on family farms, then slaughtered and eaten locally. Fruits and vegetables were also homegrown, and most families prepared their own food and ate meals at home. In recent years, however, the human food chain has changed markedly. Cattle and chickens are commonly raised by large agribusinesses, killed in mechanized slaughterhouses, and distributed to hundreds, even thousands, of food outlets in surrounding states. Fruits and vegetables are imported from distant states and, increasingly, distant countries where standards of sanitation and food processing are less stringent than our own. Families that prepare their own meals are becoming progressively fewer; instead, families buy pre-cooked and prepared foods, order in, or eat out.

Much of the increase in food-borne illnesses in the United States in recent years has been associated with ordering in and eating out. Many of the jobs in restaurant kitchens pay low wages and offer few or no sick-leave benefits, making it more likely that employees will come to work even when sick because they cannot afford not to. Many restaurant employees are also immigrants from countries where a large percentage of people suffer from intestinal diseases. According to one study, although fewer than 1 percent of individuals among the general public host a disease-carrying intestinal para-site, "in restaurants that have triggered food-borne outbreaks, up to 18 percent of food handlers have been shown to suffer intestinal infections." Contami-nation of food by an infected food handler can occur in a myriad of ways, as illustrated by a worker "who used his bare hands and arms to stir 76 liters of butter-cream frosting, an unconventional culinary technique."[1]

Some increase in food-borne illnesses has come about because of chang-ing dietary patterns. For example, raw fish, in the form of sushi or sashimi, has become popular in the United States. Fish carry more than fifty types of parasites, most of which are killed with adequate cooking. The most common infections spring from a worm called *Diphyllobothrium latum*, which causes a persistent infection characterized by diarrhea, weight loss, and anemia. Recently, there have been several cases of infection due to another parasite called *Anisakis simplex*. This parasite can cause abdominal pain and intestinal obstruction, sometimes leading to a misdiagnosis of intestinal tumors. The consumption of raw shellfish can also result in infection with hepatitis A or Norwalk-type viruses. We can avoid all these infections by not eating raw or undercooked seafood.

Changes in the human food chain have brought about many new oppor-tunities for animal microbes to cause food-borne illnesses. Not all food-borne illnesses, of course, are caused by microbes that come from animals, but the vast majority of them are. Exceptions include food-borne diseases due to con-tamination with organisms from human feces, the cause of the outbreak of hepatitis A among more than five hundred restaurant patrons who in 2003 ate contaminated green onions at a restaurant in Pennsylvania.[2]

A measure of the importance of animal microbes in causing food-borne illnesses in the United States is the Emerging Infections Program's Foodborne Diseases Active Surveillance Network, maintained by the Centers for Dis-ease Control and Prevention (CDC).[3] CDC estimates that seventy-six million

Americans contract food-borne illnesses each year, and it maintains ongoing surveys of ten microbes thought to be important causes of these illnesses. Nine of the microbes surveyed by CDC come from animals; they are *Campylobacter, Listeria, Salmonella, Escherichia coli* 0157, *Yersinia, Shigella, Cryptosporidium, Cyclospora*, and hemolytic uremic syndrome. The origin of the tenth, *Vibrio*, is not known.

Typhoid Mary, Salmonella, and Chickens

In 1915, New York health authorities banished Mary Mallon, an Irish immigrant cook, to a cottage on a small island off Manhattan, because she was infected with the bacteria *Salmonella typhi*. Although asymptomatic herself, she had caused nine typhoid outbreaks, with fifty-four cases and four deaths, by inadvertently infecting the food and water other people ingested. By the time she was banished, Mary Mallon was widely known to the public as Typhoid Mary. She remained on the island until she died in 1938.

Salmonella typhi is unusual in being one of the only serotypes among the over 2,500 known salmonella serotypes that have specifically adapted to humans. Although *Salmonella typhi* almost certainly was originally transmitted to humans from reptiles or birds, which are thought to be the origin of all salmonella, it acquired an ability to be transmitted directly from human to human, usually by contaminated food or water. That is why Mary Mallon's profession as a cook made her so dangerous.

Typhoid epidemics occurred frequently in U.S. cities in the nineteenth century. In Philadelphia, for example, an 1899 epidemic killed 948 people. During the Spanish-American War, typhoid was rampant among U.S. troops and killed seven times more soldiers than were killed by bullets.[4] Even today, *Salmonella typhi* causes twelve million illnesses worldwide each year and is an important cause of death in such countries as Indonesia, Nigeria, and India. *Salmonella typhi* thus continues to serve as an important reminder of what salmonella serotypes can do if they adapt to humans.

Fortunately, the vast majority of the known serotypes of salmonella have not yet adapted to humans and cause human disease only when they are acquired from infected chickens or eggs. Salmonella bacteria are the single largest cause of death among the known causes of food-borne illness in the United States.[5] Of the estimated 76 million Americans who develop food-borne illnesses each year, 325,000 are hospitalized and approximately 5,000, mostly elderly, die. Between 1976 and 1995, the incidence of salmonella infections increased eightfold in the United States, and even more sharply in England and other industrialized countries.[6]

Clinically, food-borne salmonella infections may vary from mild to severe. After an incubation period of one-half to three days, the infected person develops fever, abdominal pain, and severe diarrhea, which, untreated, may last for four to five days. Occasional cases develop complications such as pneumonia, endocarditis of the heart valves, pyelonephritis of the kidney, osteomyelitis of bones, arthritis of joints, or an abscess in virtually any organ. Such complications occur most commonly in the elderly, with death rates from salmonella in nursing homes estimated to be forty to seventy times higher than in the general population.[7] Newborn children are also at high risk from complications of salmonella infections, and outbreaks of salmonella infections have occurred in newborn nurseries with devastating consequences.[8] Overall, the outcome of salmonella food-borne infections is estimated as follows: 94 percent of individuals recover without medical care; 5 percent visit a physician; 0.5 percent are hospitalized; and 0.05 percent die.[9]

A disturbing recent development in human salmonella infections are reports of increasing antibiotic resistance to some salmonella serotypes. *Salmonella Newport*, for example, has been found to be "resistant to at least nine of 17 antimicrobials tested," including the antibiotic most commonly used to treat serious infections in children. A summary of such cases noted that "antimicrobial-resistant salmonella infections have been associated with an increased hospitalization rate, morbidity, and mortality."[10] A study in Denmark, for example, reported that individuals infected with a salmonella serotype resistant to quinolone antibiotics had "a mortality rate 10.3 times higher than the general population."[11] It is likely that the increase in resistance to antibiotics is due to the widespread administration of antibiotics to animals in the food chain.[12] Given the broad human exposure to salmonella bacteria, antibiotic-resistant strains pose a significant risk of future major outbreaks of disease. This development provides another example of how the management of animals used as food can affect human health.

Episodes of food-borne salmonella infections in which many people become sick are much more likely to come to public attention than are individual infections. In fact, nobody really knows how many cases of salmonellosis occur each year, because most cases are relatively mild and attributed simply to "food poisoning." It has been estimated that twenty to one hundred cases of salmonella infection go unreported for every reported case.[13] Examples of salmonella outbreaks include 688 inmates in the South Carolina prison system who in February 2001 developed severe abdominal cramps, nausea, vomiting, and diarrhea after eating tuna salad made with eggs contaminated with *Salmonella enteritidis*. Four months later in North Carolina, fifty-one persons became similarly affected after eating contaminated eggs. These were merely two of the 677 multiple-person outbreaks of salmonellosis reported in the United States between 1990 and 2001. These outbreaks alone resulted in 23,366 illnesses, 1,988 hospitalizations, and thirty-three deaths.[14]

The variety of egg products that have been linked to salmonellosis outbreaks is impressive. Scrambled eggs were the cause of outbreaks at a British prison[15] and at a restaurant chain's breakfast bar.[16] Egg sandwiches led to an outbreak at a wedding reception, and scotch eggs produced an outbreak in a hospital.[17] Hollandaise and béarnaise sauces produced illness in seventy-three individuals who had eaten at a Tennessee restaurant one evening.[18] Homemade ice cream sickened sixty-three out of seventy-five individuals at a charity bridge tournament, while an almond parfait dessert caused illness in 381 conference attendees at a hotel.[19] All five children in one family became ill with salmonellosis after eating chocolate mousse; the mousse had been prepared by one of the children at school "in a domestic science lesson."[20]

In fact, Salmonellosis outbreaks have been linked to almost every product in which eggs are used — omelets, eggnog, Caesar salad, custard, meringue pies, French toast, tartare sauce, asparagus egg sauce, quiche, lasagna, and stuffed pasta. One of the larger *Salmonella enteritidis* outbreaks, affecting more than four hundred people in the Midwest, was caused not directly by eggs but rather by an ice cream mix that had become contaminated with the bacteria "by hauling it in a tanker improperly cleaned after carrying a load of unpasteurized liquid eggs."[21]

Although *Salmonella enteritidis* has been the principal salmonella serotype implicated in recent outbreaks caused by eggs, other serotypes may also lead to outbreaks. *Salmonella heidelberg*, for example, was the cause of an outbreak among 121 patients in a California hospital; they had all eaten tapioca pudding to which raw egg whites had been added. *Salmonella heidelberg* was also the cause of "a large outbreak of salmonellosis occurring among 700 University of Utah students who attended a sorority luncheon."[22]

Salmonella typhimurium is, after *Salmonella enteritidis*, the salmonella serotype that causes the most egg-related outbreaks of disease. For example, 187 students at a college in Washington state became ill after eating chocolate meringue pie contaminated with this bacteria.[23] And in a politically noteworthy outbreak, many of the seven hundred guests at a social function in England's House of Lords became sick after eating "a variety of dishes made with mayonnaise containing fresh shell eggs" contaminated with *Salmonella typhimurium*.[24]

Accounts of egg-related salmonella infections often note that the eggs were undercooked or added raw, as in eggnogs. Experiments have shown that salmonella bacteria remains viable in eggs cooked sunny-side up or "over easy," as well as in boiled or fried eggs in which the yolk remains liquid.[25] Other experiments have shown that "cooking eggs longer than usual — boiling for seven minutes, poaching for five minutes, and frying on each side for three minutes—was necessary to destroy salmonella that was artificially inoculated into yolks." On the other hand, "no duration of frying 'sunnyside' (not turned) eggs was sufficient to kill all the salmonella."[26] The temperature of the egg prior to cooking also makes a difference; eggs taken directly from a refrigerator require longer cooking to reach a temperature that kills the salmonella.

Outbreaks of salmonellosis caused by chickens or other poultry are less frequently reported than outbreaks caused by eggs. The main reason for the discrepancy in reporting probably has to do with how eggs and chicken are most commonly served. For example, one church social may include with its dinner offerings five pieces of infected chicken, while another church social may include five infected eggs. Among the one hundred guests at the former, five eat the individual chicken pieces and become sick a day or two later, but people are not likely to connect the illness of these five people to the church social or to any specific food. At the other church social, however, the infected eggs are used to make homemade ice cream and forty people become sick. This outbreak is much more likely to be noticed, reported, and linked to the infected eggs. Infected chicken meat is most likely to be noted as a cause of an outbreak of salmonellosis when it is used in a chicken salad and consumed by many people.

In a study in England of 1,426 food-borne outbreaks of all infectious intestinal diseases, 11 percent were caused by salmonella-contaminated poultry, approximately three-quarters of which were chickens and the remainder turkeys and ducks. Among the salmonella serotypes in the poultry outbreaks, two-thirds were caused by *Salmonella enteritidis*. As in the case of eggs, undercooking the chicken or turkey appeared to be associated with increased exposure to salmonella.[27] Undercooking may occur, for example, when poultry is stuffed and then cooked at a low temperature. Precooked chickens purchased at stores have also been indicted in some outbreaks.

Salmonellosis may also be caused by the cross-contamination of other foods by salmonella-infected eggs or poultry, which can occur when kitchen utensils are not properly washed between the preparation of different foods. An example was an outbreak of salmonellosis among 102 individuals associated with a university hospital. The cause of the outbreak was traced to vanilla pudding that was apparently contaminated when it was made "in direct spatial and temporal association with the preparation of a turkey."[28]

Salmonella can also be transmitted by foods washed with water contaminated with these microbes. A recent outbreak of *Salmonella Newport* infection resulted in illness in at least seventy-eight individuals in thirteen states; fifteen were hospitalized, and two died. The outbreak was traced to the eating of contaminated mangos that came from a farm in Brazil. The source of contamination was water used in a new infusion process carried out at the farm in an attempt to remove the larvae of the Mediterranean fruit fly before exporting the mangos to the United States.[29] This is an example of how an attempt to remove one hazard can lead to new, and unexpected, hazards.

Finally, salmonellosis can be transmitted directly from chickens or other poultry when humans merely handle live birds. In 1999, outbreaks of salmonellosis occurred among children in two states. Upon investigation, it was found that the children had handled baby chicks or ducklings, many of which had been given to them as presents at Easter. The report of the outbreak noted that "one child kept young birds in his bedroom and another carried chicks inside his jacket."[30] In 1991, a similar outbreak of sixteen cases of salmonellosis caused by *Salmonella hadar* occurred among children with pet ducklings in northeastern states. "In all homes, ducklings were initially kept inside; in a least three, they were allowed to run free. In one home, a duckling lived in the bathtub where children bathed."[31]

There are several reasons for the increasing incidence of salmonella infections in the United States, including improved reporting of cases. The increasing practices of buying prepared and precooked foods and of eating out also account for some of the increase. The largest reason for the increasing incidence of salmonella infections, however, is the greater mechanization of the poultry business.

In the United States, poultry production is big business. In 2001, 85.7 billion eggs and 8.4 billion chickens were sold. On a per capita basis, every man, woman, and child consumes the equivalent of three hundred eggs and thirty chickens per year. Approximately two-thirds of the eggs are sold as shell eggs, and the rest processed as egg products in such foods as pasta, ice cream, cake mixes, and bakery products.

Large egg producers have highly automated facilities in which up to eighty thousand hens lay eggs. In the 1970s, in an attempt to increase egg production, efforts were undertaken to eradicate two serotypes of salmonella, *Salmonella gallinarum* and *Salmonella pullorum*, that affect chickens and other poultry. These serotypes do not affect humans but cause diarrhea and other illnesses in poultry, leading to decreased egg production. In severe epidemics, these bacteria have been known to kill entire flocks of chickens.[32] *Salmonella enteritidis* is closely related to these two serotypes, and in fact, studies suggest that all three serotypes evolved from a common ancestor.[33] As *Salmonella gallinarum* and *Salmonella pullorum*, which do not cause human disease, were eradicated from chickens, *Salmonella enteritidis*, which does cause human disease, took their place.[34] *Salmonella enteritidis* in very young chicks may cause symptoms, but in older chickens it is asymptomatic. Thus, an entire flock of chickens may be infected with this bacteria, with no outward sign to indicate potential problems for humans.

Chickens infected with *Salmonella enteritidis* may transmit the infection to humans through their eggs or their meat. Infection of the eggs may occur through cracks in the eggs once they have been laid if they come into contact with chicken feces or other infected material. More ominously, *Salmonella enteritidis* may be passed from the infected chicken to the egg yolk or white even before the egg is laid.[35] Thus, you can have an infected but completely healthy-looking chicken that lays infected but completely normal-looking eggs.

Eggs may also become cross contaminated during processing if the shell is cracked. Poor refrigeration allows the bacteria to multiply, making it more likely that human disease will occur if the egg is eaten raw or undercooked. Although eggs are dated for sale by retailers, the U.S. Department of Agriculture has reported that "eggs are occasionally removed from retail establishments when they are within a few days of the expiration or sell-by date stamped on the carton and returned to the processing plant," where they are given a new expiration date.[36] Such a practice would give bacteria in the egg additional time to multiply. A 1998 U.S. Department of Agriculture report, "*Salmonella Enteritidis* Risk Assessment," estimated that approximately 2.3 million eggs sold that year were infected with salmonella and thus potentially capable of causing human disease.[37] The infection rate would thus be one egg in every twenty-eight thousand.

Chickens themselves may become infected with salmonella in a variety of ways. The bacteria may be introduced into the henhouse by mice, which are common carriers, or by cats used to control the mice.[38] Since humans may be infected with *Salmonella enteritidis*, they may also carry the bacteria from henhouse to henhouse.

Cross-contamination from one infected chicken to previously noninfected chickens is thought to occur during the slaughtering process. Poultry-processing plants have become highly automated, "slaughtering up to 200 birds per minute."[39] Dead chickens are put together into scalding tanks to loosen their feathers. The feathers are then plucked by mechanical fingers. Both the scalding and the plucking processes may transmit salmonella from one chicken to another. Evisceration is also done mechanically; according to one study, when one chicken was contaminated, "the next 42 birds were contaminated with the tracer bacteria and . . . there was sporadic contamination up to the 150th bird."[40]

How often are chickens contaminated with salmonella sold in the United States? A 1998 *Consumer Reports* study of a number of brands reported a 16 percent average salmonella contamination rate, with variation by brand from 4 percent ("Foster Farms") to 53 percent (several "premium" brands).[41] Since 8.4 billion chickens were sold in the United States in 2001, a 16 percent contamination rate means that 1.3 billion of them carried salmonella. A study in England reported "that 30 percent of raw chicken carcasses are contaminated with salmonella," with *Salmonella enteritidis* the most common serotype.[42]

Salmonella can reach humans from food sources in addition to eggs and chicken. The largest salmonella outbreak in the United States occurred in Illinois and Wisconsin in 1984 and affected an estimated two hundred thousand persons. The source was milk contaminated with *Salmonella typhimurium*.[43] Outbreaks of salmonellosis caused by this serotype have also been reported as caused by "food samples associated with different types of imported vegetables, spices, and seeds, including tahini, fresh and dried spices, banana leaves, and bean sprouts." Tahini, which is made from sesame seeds, is used in hummus. Cases of salmonellosis have also been reported from eating helva, a sweet made from sesame seed that is popular in the Middle East.[44]

Outbreaks of salmonellosis have also been caused by eating undercooked ground beef or beef jerky.[45] Especially disturbing for chocolate lovers was the report of eighty cases of salmonellosis caused by "Christmas-wrapped chocolate balls" contaminated by *Salmonella eastbourne*; "bacteriological testing of samples taken at the plant implicated cocoa beans as the probable source of the salmonella organisms that, in the low-moisture chocolate, were able to survive heating during production."[46] Individuals who use marijuana also have reason to worry. In 1981, an outbreak of eighty-five cases of salmonellosis was reported as caused by marijuana contaminated by *Salmonella muenchen*. The mechanism of contamination was thought to be "direct mixing of marijuana with animal feces, which might occur as a result of fertilization with untreated animal manure, inadvertent contamination during drying or storage, or simply direct adulteration with dried animal manure to increase the weight of the product."[47]

Animal Microbes That Cause Other Food-Borne Illnesses

Although salmonella is thought to be the leading cause of fatalities in the United States from food-borne illnesses, the CDC has identified five other microbes that also account for a significant number of deaths.[48] These are the bacteria that cause listeriosis, campylobacteriosis, and colitis due to *Escherichia coli*; the parasite that causes toxoplasmosis (see chapter 7); and the Norwalk viruses that cause diarrhea. The first four of these are usually transmitted from animals to humans. Norwalk viruses, the most common cause of viral diarrhea in adults, are thought to be transmitted from person to person. However, recent studies have identified strains of Norwalk viruses in farm animals, raising the possibility that these agents may also be transmitted from animals, or that animals may serve as reservoirs of infection.[49]

Although not yet a household name, listeriosis is emerging as an important food-borne illness because about one-third of human cases are fatal. It is caused by a remarkably hardy bacterium, *Listeria monocytogenes*, that can survive for up to two years in the soil. It has been identified in more than forty species of domestic mammals and twenty species of birds, including chickens, ducks, and turkeys. In sheep and goats, listeriosis is an important cause of abortion and other illnesses.

Listeriosis is transmitted from animals to humans mostly through contaminated foods. Outbreaks that involve large groups of people have been attributed to foods as diverse as cheese, pork, turkey, paté, mussels, coleslaw, and milk.[50] Individuals most likely to be infected are pregnant women, the elderly, and persons with impaired immune systems. Infection in pregnant women commonly leads to spontaneous abortion, premature birth, or serious infection of the newborn; surviving infants can have adverse long-term consequences, especially if the infection involves the brain or central nervous system. In elderly and immunocompromised individuals, listeriosis begins as a flulike illness, then may proceed to meningitis, with fever, headache, or dissemination of the bacteria throughout the body.

The mortality rate from listeriosis is notably high. An outbreak in northeastern states during the summer of 2002 led to seven deaths and three stillbirths among forty-six cases.[51] The cause of the outbreak was contamination of turkey deli meat at a poultry-processing plant in Pennsylvania. It led to the recall of 27.4 million pounds of meat, the nation's largest meat recall up to that time, as well as to public accusations that the government was not doing enough to protect the nation's food supply.[52]

Campylobacteriosis is another important but little-known food-borne infection. Recognized only twenty-five years ago, it has since been labeled "the most common form of acute infective diarrhea identified in most industrialized countries of the world."[53]

Campylobacteriosis is caused by *Campylobacter* bacteria, which are closely related to *Helicobacter* bacteria, the cause of gastric ulcers. It predominantly affects children and young adults, beginning with flulike symptoms and a fever and progressing to severe diarrhea with abdominal pain. In most cases, the illness lasts only two or three days and remits without complications. In approximately 1 percent of cases, campylobacteriosis is followed by arthritis or by the Guillain-Barré syndrome, a severe neurological illness. *Campylobacter* bacteria have also recently been linked to immunoproliferative small intestine disease, a type of lymphoma.[54]

Campylobacter bacteria are widely distributed among birds and among some domestic animals. Approximately half of all cases of campylobacteriosis come from chickens, especially those processed by poultry-processing plants, in which one infected bird may contaminate others. Contaminated chickens may spread their microbes to other foods as well; as one account notes: "It does not require much imagination to appreciate the ease with which a few hundred bacteria can be transferred from, say, a fresh broiler covered in a million bacteria to a nearby bit of salad or piece of bread."[55] Undercooked chicken or other meat, as often occurs in barbecues and fondue cooking, are especially likely to cause problems.

An unusual outbreak of campylobacteriosis in England was caused by milk bottles that were capped with only an aluminum foil cover and left on the doorstep by milk-truck drivers. Magpies and jackdaws, both of which carry *Campylobacter*, learned to peck through the caps of the milk bottles to get the milk, and thereby contaminated the milk with *Campylobacter*. This problem was solved by putting more substantial caps on the milk bottles.

The third bacterial disease identified by the CDC as responsible for a significant number of food-borne illness-associated deaths in the United States is diarrheal disease caused by the *Escherichia coli* and *Shigella* complex. Although these were originally believed to be separate bacterial families, we now know that they are part of a single family.[56] The most lethal member of this group is *Escherichia coli* serotype 0157, which has been responsible for several outbreaks of severe diarrheal disease.

Escherichia coli in humans may cause mild diarrhea, severe diarrhea with bloody stools (dysentery), or a hemolytic uremic syndrome (HUS) that is a leading cause of kidney failure in children. At least 5 percent of children with HUS die, and a third more have chronic kidney problems such as hypertension.

Escherichia coli bacteria are widely distributed in cattle, most of which are asymptomatic carriers. Transmission to humans occurs primarily through undercooked beef, particularly in the form of beefburgers, or through unpasteurized milk, but it may occur by any exposure to food or water contaminated with cattle feces. In Scotland, for example, a 1996 outbreak caused by contaminated meat from a local butcher affected more than 400 persons, of which 151 were admitted to hospitals and 18 died.[57] A 1996 outbreak in Japan affected more than 6,000 schoolchildren, and 102 of them developed kidney disease with a HUS.[58] In the United States, thirty-seven children developed the hemolytic uremic syndrome after eating beefburgers at a Jack in the Box restaurant in the Seattle area. Half of the children also had abnormalities in other organs, including the heart, lung, pancreas, intestinal tract, and central nervous system, and three of the children died. Further investigation revealed that this was part of a three-state outbreak comprising 501 cases of disease resulting in 301 hospitalizations. The main source of illness appeared to be undercooked beefburgers.[59] Similar outbreaks have been reported in other areas of the country; in some cases, the outbreaks were not recognized as such until they were investigated by public health officials.[60]

Escherichia coli may occasionally be transmitted to humans from other animals, including pigs, goats, and sheep. It may also contaminate a variety of other foods that may then cause outbreaks of human disease. For example, in 1997, contaminated alfalfa sprouts were responsible for an outbreak in Virginia among forty-eight persons, eleven of whom were hospitalized. Similarly, a 1998 outbreak in North Carolina that affected 142 people was attributed to contaminated coleslaw in a restaurant, and a 1999 outbreak in Nebraska that affected 72 people was due to contaminated lettuce in a restaurant.[61]

The Message from Mad Cows

On December 23, 2003, U.S. secretary of agriculture Ann Veneman called a news conference to announce the diagnosis of bovine spongiform encephalopathy (BSE), popularly known as mad cow disease, in the first U.S. cow. Seven months earlier, BSE had been reported in a Canadian cow, so the announcement should have been expected, especially when it was revealed that the U.S. cow had come from a Canadian herd. Even so, stocks in beef-related companies fell sharply, other nations shut their doors to U.S. beef exports, and thousands of Americans who had possibly eaten beef from the infected cow worried.

At the news conference, Veneman said: "The risk to human health is extremely low. . . . I plan to serve beef for my Christmas dinner, and we remain confident in the safety of our food supply."[62] Veneman's assurances were reminiscent of those provided in 1989 by John Gummer, the British minister of agriculture, during an outbreak of BSE in England. At that time, there had been no proven cases of BSE having been transmitted from cows to humans. Gummer, accompanied by his four-year-old daughter, appeared on television to publicly assure people that eating beef was safe, as the two of them were shown eating large beefburgers.

Such assurances were revealed to have been overly optimistic in 1995, when a young Royal Air Force cadet became the first known human victim of BSE. By mid-2004, a total of 146 British citizens and eleven individuals in other countries had died; all were thought to have gotten BSE by eating contaminated beef. In addition, testing of lymphatic tissue randomly taken from

British citizens during routine removal of tonsils and appendices suggested that as many as 3,800 other individuals are harboring the prions thought to cause BSE;[63] how many of them will eventually develop disease is unknown. The British epidemic of BSE among cattle was eventually controlled by slaughtering four million of them. A prominent victim of the BSE epidemic was the Conservative Party, which went down to resounding defeat, in part because of its perceived mishandling of the BSE epidemic.

The prions thought to cause BSE are strange and poorly understood microbes. They are bits of protein that contain no genetic material—neither DNA nor RNA—and yet are able to reproduce within cells and cause disease. They are not bacteria, viruses, or protozoa but rather variant proteins that function as infectious agents by becoming misfolded, thus changing their structure and clinical properties. Prions attack brain tissue, producing small holes that give the brain the appearance of a sponge, when examined under a microscope after death. This gives rise to the official name of prion diseases, spongiform encephalopathies. Prions are also strange insofar as they may take years to cause symptoms after they have entered the human body. For many cases of human BSE, this latent period is thought to be ten years or longer, and for other human prion diseases, the latent period may be as long as twenty years.

Symptoms of human prion disease include mental changes, memory loss, involuntary movements, seizures, and an inevitable progression to dementia and death. There is no known treatment. The best-studied human prion disease is Creutzfeldt-Jakob disease (CJD), which affects approximately one person in every million; human BSE is officially referred to as "variant CJD." CJD may be transmitted from one infected individual after death to another individual through the transplantation of postmortem brain tissue, such as dural grafts or pituitary growth hormone, or through corneal transplants. CJD may also arise spontaneously, and there is thought to be a genetic predisposition to acquiring it. Researchers have suggested that some "spontaneous" cases of CJD may in fact be caused by a person's having eaten beef from cows infected by BSE; if this is true, then variant CJD obtained from BSE-infected cows and "spontaneous" CJD may be variants of the same disease.

Another human prion disease is kuru, which was until recently endemic in the highlands of Papua New Guinea. It was transmitted from person to person through the eating of brains of dead relatives as a part of local funeral rituals.

The transmission of BSE between cattle, and from cattle to humans, is a direct consequence of modern methods of raising and slaughtering cattle. For thousands of years, cattle were raised on small farms where calves were nursed by their mothers. Such bucolic scenes have been largely replaced by giant agribusinesses where "for years calves have been fed cow's blood instead of milk, and cattle feed has been allowed to contain composted wastes from chicken coops, including feathers, spilled feed, and even feces."[64]

Furthermore, for many years, calves and cattle were fed meat- and-bone meal, which is made from dead cattle. Meat-and-bone meal is a product of rendering, which is essentially the boiling of animal carcasses to obtain fat and protein. Although rules now prohibit the feeding of cattle-derived meat-and-bone meal to other cattle, it still is commonly fed to chickens and pigs. When the chickens and pigs die, they may, in turn, be rendered, and the product fed to cattle. It is a widely used system of high-tech barnyard cannibalism. Meat-and-bone meal is also a common ingredient in pet foods.

The main danger of meat-and-bone meal is that it may contain tissue from the central nervous system, including the brain, spinal cord, or nerves, the main tissues thought to contain prions. Meat-and-bone meal made from a single animal infected with BSE can theoretically infect hundreds of others when they ingest the meat-and-bone meal. The BSE epidemic among British cattle in the 1980s and 1990s was, in fact, caused by an inadvertent change in the process by which meat-and-bone meal was being made, making it more likely that prions would be passed on.[65]

The transmission of BSE from infected cattle to humans is also a consequence of mechanized advanced meat-recovery systems that try to recover every possible ounce of meat. These systems sometimes also recover tissue from the brain or spinal cord, or other nerve tissue. Testing by the Department of Agriculture in 2002 found that 35 percent of advanced meat-recovery systems included such tissue.[66] This tissue may then become incorporated into ground beef, sausage, bologna, salami, hot dogs, pizza meat toppings, taco fillings, and similar foods. If a BSE-infected cow happens to be included, infective meat may be distributed widely within days of its processing. As a general rule, eating whole beef, such as steak or roast beef, is safer than eating ground beef, such as beefburger meat, since the latter is more likely to have tissue mixed with it that may include prions.

The first reported case of BSE in U.S. cattle stimulated changes in the beef industry. Until then, less than 1 percent of the thirty-five million cattle slaughtered each year in the United States was tested for BSE; that percentage has now increased. Regulations were also tightened regarding the composition of meat-and-bone meal and the functioning of advanced meat-recovery systems. Whether these changes will protect the U.S. food chain from the transmission of animal prion diseases will not be known for a number of years. Because of the long latent period between humans' becoming infected with prions and the onset of symptoms, it is difficult to assess the effectiveness of such prevention programs.

Other prion diseases of animals include scrapie in sheep and transmissible mink encephalopathy, but these diseases are not known to be transmitted to humans. Recently, however, a prion disease of deer and elk, chronic wasting disease (CWD), has come under scrutiny. CWD has spread progressively across western states and caused concern among deer hunters, many of whom serve venison to their families.[67] To date, there has been no proven transmission of CWD to humans, although there are reports of Creutzfeldt-Jakob disease in deer hunters who have regularly eaten venison.[68]

In summary, of all the food-borne diseases transmitted from animals to humans, BSE is the most publicized and most feared. This is ironic, since the only person in the United States who has died from BSE became infected while living in England. The chances of dying from BSE are considerably lower than the chances of being struck by lightning. Meanwhile, hundreds of Americans die each year from salmonellosis, listeriosis, campylobacteriosis, and colitis due to *Escherichia coli*.

The truly worrisome aspect of prion diseases, including BSE and CWD, is that so little is known about what prions really do. BSE has been transmitted through contaminated food that contains beef protein to nonhuman primates.[69] BSE has also been transmitted to cats by contaminated pet food.[70] In one especially disturbing case, both a cat and its owner simultaneously developed fatal Creutzfeldt-Jakob disease, although the authors of the report noted that the cases could have resulted from "horizontal transmission in either direction, infection from an unknown common source, or the chance occurrence of two sporadic forms."[71] Mice, hamsters, and raccoons are susceptible to prion disease when artificially injected.[72] There are also suggestions that prion diseases can be passed from infected mothers to their fetuses.[73] A study showed that some animals may be infected with prion disease, have no symptoms, but still be capable of infecting other animals.[74] Especially worrisome was a study that showed that prions may become more pathogenic when passed from one animal species to another.[75]

Given the many unknowns, it would appear prudent to be conservative in establishing safeguards for our meat supply. The steps taken following the first U.S. case of BSE in cattle to test more cattle for BSE, keep sick cattle out of the food chain, and make meat-recovery systems safer are steps in the right direction. But are they enough?

9

C H A P T E R

Microbes from the Modern Food Chain

Lessons from SARS, Influenza, and Bird Flu

The bottom line is that humans have to think about how they treat their animals, how they farm them, and how they market them — basically the whole relationship between the animal kingdom and the human kingdom is coming under stress.

PETER CORDINGLY, World Health Organization

THAT ANIMAL microbes can be transmitted to humans when humans eat the meat, milk, or eggs of infected animals is widely known. Less widely known is that animal microbes can also be transmitted to humans as a consequence of the modern food chain. As our food chain has become more complex and commercialized, opportunities have increased for new microbes to emerge and old microbes to undergo mutations. Such changes may produce new and serious threats to human health, as SARS, influenza, and bird flu (a form of influenza) illustrate.

Wet Markets and SARS

In the spring of 2003, the city of Toronto was virtually shut down. The World Health Organization and CDC issued travel advisories that warned visitors not to go there, and hotel operators lost $125 million in revenue. The cause of the shutdown was an epidemic of SARS (severe acute respiratory syndrome) that killed 24 individuals in Toronto and 910 worldwide. Some people wore masks in public, a phenomenon not seen since the 1918–1919 influenza pandemic.

The origin of the SARS epidemic was live animal markets, widely referred to as *wet markets*, in southern China.[1] Permanent large open markets in cities such as Guangzhou and Shenzhen sell a variety of live animals that are purchased as food. The animals include chickens, ducks, geese, pigeons, doves, turtles, dogs, cats, crabs, and other seafood, as well as exotic animals such as palm civets, raccoon dogs, and ferret badgers. One observer noted that "everything that's vaguely edible is for sale."[2] Such markets often look as if Noah's ark had just been offloaded there, with hundreds of metal cages stacked two and three high packed with animals, vendors sometimes napping on top of the cages, and masses of people circulating among the cages, looking, coughing, sneezing, drinking, and eating. For animal microbes looking for new homes, wet markets are paradise.

Following the outbreak of SARS in 2003, the causative agent was rapidly ascertained to be a coronavirus. Coronaviruses are known to infect dogs, cats, cows, horses, pigs, chickens, turkeys, mice, and rats, as well as humans. In humans, one type of coronavirus is a frequent cause of the common cold. Coronaviruses are also known to selectively cross species barriers, such as a coronavirus of cows that can also infect chickens but not turkeys. The coronavirus responsible for the SARS outbreak was a novel type not previously seen, and molecular studies suggested that it had probably evolved from another coronavirus shortly before the outbreak.[3]

The specific animal origin of the SARS coronavirus, at this writing, has yet to be determined. Palm civets, an animal related to the mongoose, are commonly sold in the Chinese markets as food, and many of them were found to be carrying the virus. On the basis of that finding, Chinese authorities ordered the killing of approximately ten thousand palm civets being raised on farms for sale to the markets. However, when a second outbreak of SARS occurred in 2004, one victim had been trapping rats in his apartment, and some of the rats tested positive for SARS.[4] Rats had also been suspected of playing a role in the original epidemic.[5] The question of identifying the definitive reservoir of the SARS virus was further confused when mice, ferrets, cats, foxes, and monkeys were all shown capable of becoming infected under certain conditions.

The SARS epidemic demonstrated that the SARS virus has the potential to spread very rapidly from person to person and to kill approximately 9 percent of those infected. Transmission of the virus may occur through respiratory droplets, as when a person coughs or sneezes, or through urine, feces, or even sweat; thus, it is possible to get SARS merely by touching an infected person.[6] With the assistance of air travel, SARS spread to thirty countries on five continents within a few weeks.[7] Especially worrisome was that some infected individuals, called "super-spreaders," appear to be highly infectious and capable of transmitting the virus to large numbers of people, whereas other people may carry the SARS virus and show few, if any, symptoms.[8] Also, between its appearance in 2003 and its reappearance in smaller outbreaks in 2004, the SARS virus underwent minor changes, producing a marked increase in its ability to infect humans.[9]

Fish Farming and Influenza

Influenza is not usually considered a disease associated with modern food chains, but in fact, it is. If not for the system of fish farming in southern China, with its juxtaposition of ducks, fish, pigs, and humans, influenza as a disease would probably not have emerged to become a major source of epidemics around the world.

Any understanding of influenza must begin with ducks, which, along with other aquatic birds, are the natural reservoir for influenza viruses. Herons, gulls, terns, shearwaters, guillemots, and sandpipers are also infected with influenza viruses, but their role in spreading influenza to other species is not clear. Ducks are the aquatic species of interest, because ducks, domesticated approximately four thousand years ago, have had extensive contact with humans. Twenty-three of the known twenty-four subtypes of influenza A are found in ducks, with the remaining subtype found in gulls and other shorebirds. According to influenza expert Robert Webster, there is "a vast reservoir of influenza A viruses in aquatic birds."[10]

Ducks and other aquatic birds have probably been infected with influenza viruses for millions of years. By contrast, the current strains of influenza viruses that infect humans emerged only eight thousand years ago.[11] Farmers who raise domestic fowl have long observed the immunity of ducks to the symptoms of influenza, even when ducks are raised in the same farmyards with chickens and turkeys that may be experiencing severe symptoms of the disease.[12] Molecular studies of the virus also suggest that the avian influenza viral proteins are relatively stable as compared to the proteins in human strains of influenza. If ducks had not been domesticated, we might not even be aware of the existence of influenza A viruses.

Ducks were probably first domesticated in China and are most numerous there. Rice is also cultivated in China. Ducks are useful in rice growing, since they feed on the weeds and insects in the rice paddy but leave the rice alone. Ducks can also be used for their eggs and meat. It has been estimated that there are more domestic ducks than people in China, especially in the southern provinces, where rice growing is widespread.

Alongside rice fields and ducks in southern China, fish farming also developed. The fish are reared in natural or artificial ponds and used for food. As fish farming developed, it was discovered that fertilizing the ponds with animal feces produced bigger fish. The feces stimulate the growth of plankton, which is then eaten by the fish. Pigs, chickens, and ducks have traditionally been used as sources for excrement to fertilize the fishponds. In some cases, the feces are collected, dried, and then broadcast widely over the pond. In other cases, pigs, chickens, or ducks are confined in cages suspended over the fishpond, so that their feces drop directly into the water. Such systems have become increasingly elaborate, as is one described in Thailand, where "wide use is made of pig-hen-fish culture: the hens are in cages above the pigs which consume hen feces, and the pigs are in pens directly above the fish ponds into which they defecate."[13] In recent years, fish farming has become more widespread throughout Southeast Asia and is often referred to as aquaculture, or the "Blue Revolution." In 1970, a World Aquaculture Society was formed; there is an Asia-Pacific Regional Research and Training Center for Integrated Fish Farming in China; and manuals such as "Integrated Fish Farming in China" are available. Fish farming is said to have "grown at over 10 percent annually during the past decade," and "within a decade it may overtake world beef production."[14]

The juxtaposition of fishponds with ducks, pigs, chickens, other animals, and humans is a unique combination that leads to rapid changes in the influenza virus. Influenza A viruses consist of eight separate genetic units of RNA. Each of the eight genetic units in turn encodes multiple units of messenger RNA, and these are constantly changing. Mutations in the RNA genome lead to alterations in the viral proteins, with resulting changes in the ability of the virus to replicate, cause disease, and escape detection by the host immune system. This process produces a slow change called *genetic drift*. Occasionally, one of the eight genetic units is completely replaced, producing a much more rapid change called *genetic shift*. Insofar as the genetic drift or genetic shift produces changes in the two key molecules—hemagglutinin (H) and neuraminidase (N)—that lie in the protein coat of the virus, the influenza virus is no longer as recognizable to cells that previously could produce antibodies against it.

This constant change in the influenza virus is why many individuals must get a flu shot every year. Last year's flu shot was made to elicit antibodies against the specific array of H and N antigens that existed in the virus at that time. However, during the year, the antigen array often changes, so that last year's flu shot may be only partly effective in eliciting antibodies against this year's virus. When an entire genetic unit is replaced, as occurs in genetic shift, last year's flu shot may elicit almost no antibodies at all. Genetic drift and genetic shift are mechanisms influenza viruses use to continuously adapt to new host cells and thereby avoid antibodies left over from past infections or past vaccines.

It is now thought that genetic shift of influenza viruses occurs when two or more viruses infect one animal, thereby allowing the genetic components to recombine and form a new strain. Pigs are unusual insofar as they can become simultaneously infected with more than one strain of influenza virus. One study, for example, found that 14 percent of the pigs studied were infected with two strains of influenza virus.[15] This is the main mechanism by which genetic shift is thought to take place, bringing about the replacement of a hemaggluti-nin (H) or neuraminidase (N) surface antigen by a new antigen. Pigs are thus like mixing bowls for influenza viruses, "the leading contender for the role of intermediate host for reassortment" of the genetic segments.[16]

Fish farming as practiced in Southeast Asia presents ideal circumstances for the genetic reassortment of influenza viruses. Ducks, both wild and domes-tic, regularly swim in the fishponds that have been fertilized with pig feces. They drink the water and also take in the water through their cloaca. Ducks also release water and feces into the water, along with whatever influenza vi-ruses they happen to be carrying. Pigs are given that same water to drink and thereby ingest the influenza viruses. The pigs may also be fed the carcasses of dead ducks. No longer confined to ducks, the influenza viruses are provided with repeated and prolonged access to pigs and other animals that drink the pond water. When a new strain of virus evolves in its passage between ducks, pigs, and humans, its widespread distribution is further guaranteed by wild ducks that land on the fish pond, drink the water, and migrate thousands of miles to distribute the virus to other bodies of water.

It should be emphasized that it is the juxtaposition of domestic ducks, which are the reservoir for influenza viruses, to pigs and humans that leads to the development of new influenza strains. In the absence of ducks, fish farm-ing would not pose a threat. Similarly, where ducks are abundant but other animals are largely absent, there is also little threat. For example, many Cana-dian lakes at which large numbers of wild ducks collect during the summer months are said to be "a veritable witches' brew of avian influenza."[17] But be-cause no pigs or other domesticated animals drink the water from those lakes, there is apparently no reassortment of influenza genes and thus no emergence of new influenza strains.

Given the antiquity of fish farming in China and what is now known about the origins of human influenza, it is not surprising that epidemics of the disease have occurred for several centuries. An epidemic in London in 1562 that was probably influenza was described as "a new disease that is common in this towne . . . which passed also throughe [the queen's] whole courte, neither sparinge leaders, ladies nor damoysells. . . . There is no appearance of danger, nor manie that die of the disease, except some olde folks." An epidemic in 1781 was especially severe: "In St. Petersburg 30,000 fell ill each day, in Rome two-thirds of the population were attacked, and in Munich three-quarters. . . . All reports state that it started in China in the autumn."[18]

Medical historians agree that epidemics of influenza have increased in the past two centuries, perhaps as a result of more fish farming and improved transportation of the virus. Pandemics occurred in 1802, 1830, 1847, and 1857. The especially severe pandemic of 1889 began in central Asia and was thus named the "Asiatic flu"; it affected up to half the population in some European cities, killing up to 1 percent of those affected. Young adults were especially affected, a harbinger of what was to come three decades later.

The influenza pandemic of 1918–1919 demonstrated to the world the lethal potential of new influenza strains. The pandemic is estimated to have killed worldwide more than twenty million people and "ranks among the worst disasters in human history."[19] According to Alfred Crosby's definitive history of the pandemic, "nothing else — no infection, no war, no famine — has ever killed so many in as short a period."[20] Approximately 550,000 died in the United States, more than the number of Americans killed in World War I, World War II, the Korean War, and the war in Vietnam combined.

The earliest manifestations of the pandemic occurred in Spain in the spring of 1918. Because it was first reported there, it acquired the name "Spanish flu," but its real origin is unknown. A medical commission concluded that it had begun in Turkestan, while others asserted that it had been brought to Europe by Chinese workers hired to dig trenches for the Allied forces. An analysis of the influenza virus strain responsible for the pandemic has established that it first infected humans between 1900 and 1915 and had been quietly circulating for several years before it developed into an epidemic.[21]

The pandemic arrived in the United States in August. In Boston, hundreds of sailors awaiting deployment to Europe developed influenza in the crowded barracks, and civilians began following suit in early September. Alarmingly, many of these young and otherwise healthy young men were dying, which was not supposed to occur with influenza. The deaths caused concern within the medical community, and the Boston stock market was closed. But it was difficult to get the public's attention: In France, 896,000 U.S. troops were preparing to attack the German lines, and at Fenway Park, Babe Ruth and the Boston Red Sox were preparing to play the Chicago Cubs in the World Series. In Boston schools, girls jumped rope to a new song:

I had a little bird
And its name was Enza.
I opened the window
And in-flew-Enza.[22]

Influenza spread rapidly among the U.S. troops preparing to leave for France. At many bases in the United States, between 35 and 40 percent of the men were affected, approximately 3 percent of them fatally. At Fort Devens, Massachusetts, a physician described how the flu developed: "These men start with what appears to be an ordinary attack of . . . influenza . . . and when brought to the hospital they very rapidly develop the most viscous type of pneumonia that has ever been seen. Two hours after admission they have the mahogany spots over the cheek bones, and a few hours later you can begin to see the cyanosis extending from their ears and spreading all over the face, until it is hard to distinguish the colored men from the white. It is only a matter of a few hours then until death comes, and it is simply a struggle for air until they suffocate. It is horrible. . . . We have been averaging about 100 deaths per day."[23] At Fort Devens, "special trains" were needed to carry away the soldiers dying from influenza. Approximately four thousand soldiers and sailors died aboard troopships while being transported to Europe or shortly after landing there. Influenza's effects on U.S. troops were devastating. The U.S. Army's Eighty-eighth Division suffered 90 men killed, wounded, missing, or captured in battle, but 444 others died from influenza.[24] The high mortality rate in the 1918 epidemic, especially among young people, has never been fully explained. It is possible that secondary bacterial infections caused much of it, in which case antibiotics would have saved many lives. On the other hand, it may simply have been a very lethal strain of the virus, in which case antibiotics would not have helped.

By October 1918, influenza was spreading rapidly through the civilian population with similarly lethal effects. Philadelphia was especially hard hit, suffering approximately eleven thousand deaths. At the city morgue, dead bodies "were piled three and four deep in the corridors and in almost every room, covered only with dirty and often bloodstained sheets. . . . Six wagons and a motor truck toured the city and collected . . . corpses."[25] On October 10 in Philadelphia, 759 people died from influenza. On October 23 in New York City, 851 died. In Chicago, "trolleys were draped in black and used to collect the bodies," and funerals were restricted to a maximum of ten attendees in addition to the undertaker.[26] Washington, D.C., hospitals "stationed undertakers at their doors to remove each body as soon as death occurred to make room for another patient."[27] One anecdotal account of influenza's lethal effects told of four women who played bridge together one evening; by the next morning three were dead. Another told of a man who boarded a streetcar to go to work but died after it had gone only six blocks. In Washington, D.C., Congressman Jacob Meeker came down with the flu, whereupon he immediately married his secretary and "died a few hours later."[28]

One of the most visually striking symbols of the 1918 influenza pandemic in the United States was the use of gauze masks. Although there was no evidence that masks retarded the spread of the influenza viruses, authorities were desperate to do something, so local ordinances were passed making masks mandatory in public places and "in any place where two or more persons are congregated . . . except when partaking of meals." Surreal photographs show weddings at which everyone in attendance, including the bride and groom, is wearing a mask. A picture of a minor league baseball game shows every player and spectator wearing a mask. Pictures show masked voters casting ballots in the November 5 national election. And when news of the armistice reached the United States, there were scenes of "tens of thousands of deliriously happy, singing, masked celebrants."[29]

Many Americans opposed the wearing of masks. Called "mask slackers," they faced fines and in some cities were not allowed to board buses or streetcars. Since there appeared to be no difference in the influenza rate between those who wore masks and those who did not, however, the public grew increasingly skeptical of their value. Civil libertarians and Christian Scientists led the opposition for what came to be called the Anti-Mask League. As 1918 drew to a close, tobacconists complained that cigarette and cigar sales were down by 50 percent because people could not smoke with their masks on. Restaurant owners also said that business was down sharply, and shop owners worried that masks would discourage people from Christmas shopping. And there were practical problems. In San Francisco, the police complained that the use of masks had encouraged robberies. In Macon, Georgia, masked army medics awaited the arrival of fifteen hundred black recruits at the train station. When the black recruits descended onto the platform, they fled in terror, believing that the medics were Ku Klux Klansmen.[30]

Isolated communities in which people had been less exposed to previous influenza outbreaks, and thus had fewer antibodies to help ameliorate the new strain, were especially hard hit. The case mortality among Native Americans was 9 percent, four times the rate in U.S. cities.[31] In Nome, Alaska, 59 percent of the town's three hundred Eskimos died. In the nearby Eskimo village of Teller, 53 percent of the inhabitants died. In Teller Mission, six miles away, "85 percent of the population perished in a single week."[32]

The 1918–1919 influenza pandemic also affected many U.S. writers. Mary McCarthy was six years old and living in Seattle when her mother and father both became ill. Alarmed, the family boarded a train for their grandparents' home in Minneapolis. A conductor tried to force them off the train "at a small wooden station in the middle of the North Dakota prairie," but Mary's father, brandishing a gun, insisted that they were going to continue their journey. Five days after they arrived in Minneapolis, her father and mother were both dead. Mary and her three siblings, along with hundreds of thousands of other children, were orphans.[33]

Thomas Wolfe was a student at the University of North Carolina when he was summoned home by the onset of influenza in his brother Benjamin. Wolfe later described his brother's death in a slightly fictionalized passage in *Look Homeward, Angel*: "Ben lay upon the bed below them, drenched in light, like some enormous insect on a naturalist's table, fighting, while they looked at him, to save with his poor wasted body the life that no one could save for him. It was monstrous, brutal."[34]

In Denver, Katherine Anne Porter was a twenty-four-year-old newspaper reporter and deeply in love with her fiancé, who was going off to war. She developed influenza so severely that "the newspaper set the type for her obituary."[35] She survived, but her fiancé was afflicted by it and died shortly thereafter at his army training camp. Years later, Porter fictionalized those difficult days in *Pale Horse, Pale Rider*:

> "I wonder," said Miranda. "How did you manage to get an extension of leave?"
>
> "They just gave it," said Adam, "for no reason. The men are dying like flies out there, anyway. This funny new disease. Simply knocks you into a cocked hat."
>
> "It seems to be a plague," said Miranda, "something out of the Middle Ages. Did you ever see so many funerals, ever?[36]

Outbreaks of influenza continued to occur following the 1918–1919 disaster, but no true pandemic was seen again until 1957. Called the "Asian flu," this pandemic started in southern China and progressively spread around the world. In the United States, it was responsible for approximately sixty thousand deaths, mostly among the elderly. Another influenza pandemic, the "Hong Kong flu," swept across much of the world in 1968 and killed approximately thirty thousand Americans. In 1976, at what appeared to be the beginning of another influenza epidemic, the "swine flu" scare led to massive vaccination of the population; the epidemic never appeared, and the vaccinations themselves caused significant illness. It was a political and public health imbroglio.

The influenza pandemics of 1918, 1957, and 1968 were each the result of a genetic shift of the virus that created new strains. All three were mixtures of viruses from ducks and viruses that had adapted to pigs and to humans.

The 1918 strain was described as "a chimera of sorts: One end bore a marked resemblance to human flu sequences, the middle was strikingly similar to pig, while the other end again was human."[37] The strain of influenza virus that caused the 1957 pandemic had three genetic segments from a duck virus and five segments from a human virus, while the strain that caused the 1968 pandemic had two of the former and six of the latter.[38] Influenza experts are unanimous in predicting that another pandemic will occur, and most believe that it will appear soon.

Poultry Farming and Bird Flu

Influenza A viruses can affect chickens and other poultry, just as they can affect many other animals. Bird flu, as it is now commonly called, was previously called "fowl plague" and described a century ago; in the intervening years, outbreaks of bird flu have resulted in deaths among chickens, turkeys, and, occasionally, domestic ducks. Wild ducks and other aquatic birds, thought to be the natural reservoir for influenza viruses, are usually not affected by outbreaks of bird flu among poultry. Until recent years, poultry farming was usually done on a small scale. Now it is increasingly carried out as part of larger agribusinesses, and what were once flocks of dozens of poultry are now flocks of thousands. Thus, when bird flu strikes, it can spread more rapidly and widely.

Before 1997, there had never been reports of influenza being transmitted directly from birds to humans, since pigs were thought to be necessary as genetic mixing bowls. In 1997, during an outbreak of bird flu in Hong Kong, the influenza virus was directly transmitted from infected chickens to eighteen people, six of whom died. These first proven cases of bird flu in humans were widely considered an ominous development. The strain of influenza virus that was responsible was H5; until then, all human cases of influenza had been caused by H1, H2, or H3 strains. The 1997 outbreak suggested that chickens, like pigs, might serve as mixing vessels for the development of new influenza strains. And if new strains can occur in chickens, can they also occur in other animal species known to be infected with influenza, such as horses, cows, dogs, deer, seals, whales, monkeys, or humans?

Following the 1997 outbreak, the H5 influenza strain continued to circulate in ducks in China, but no additional human cases were reported. Then, in February 2003, two Hong Kong residents returned from a visit to southern China with bird flu, and one of them died. In December 2003, a severe epidemic of H5 (specifically H5N1) bird flu began in Korea. The virus appeared to be highly pathogenic for chickens, killing them in two or three days, with

100 percent mortality in some flocks. The H5N1 strain of virus is thought to undergo mutations rapidly and to have "a documented propensity to acquire genes from viruses infecting other animal species."[39]

The H5N1 epidemic of bird flu spread rapidly across Southeast Asia, infecting poultry in ten other countries within two months. In an effort to limit its spread, public health officials ordered the slaughter of all poultry geographically proximate to infected flocks; by mid 2004, it was estimated that more than 100 million chickens, turkeys, geese, and ducks had been killed.[40] The magnitude of the bird flu outbreak among poultry was termed "historically unprecedented."[41]

As the bird flu spread more widely, it began to infect other animals. In Thailand, several housecats became infected and died, as did a leopard in a zoo. All were thought to have been fed infected dead chickens. Then human cases were reported. Among the first thirty-seven human cases, all reported from Vietnam and Thailand, twenty-three individuals died, a mortality rate of 62 percent.[42] Almost all the victims had had direct contact with poultry, and it was assumed that the virus had spread directly from the poultry to them.

Until January 2004, there was no evidence of the spread of bird flu from person to person. (As noted in chapter 1, many microbes spread from animals to humans but then spread no further.) For a microbe originally transmitted from an animal to a human to then spread from human to human usually requires the microbe to undergo some reassortment of genes or mutations. This is a big step that most microbes, fortunately, do not take. In an editorial in the *New England Journal of Medicine*, the difference between animal-to-human transmission and animal-to-human-to-human transmission was likened to the words of the first astronaut who landed on the moon. When a microbe crosses the species barrier from animal to human, it was said to be "one small step to man." Developing the ability to spread from human to human, however, is "one giant leap to mankind."[43]

The development of an ability to be transmitted from human to human is the major fear surrounding bird flu. In January 2004, four cases of bird flu occurred in a single family immediately following a wedding. The groom and both sisters who had nursed him died, while the bride became infected but survived. Two of the four had had no known contact with poultry, and it was assumed, although not proven, that this was the first recorded person-to-person transmission.[44]

The H5N1 outbreak of bird flu and its spread to humans was not the only bad news. In 1999, an H9N2 strain of influenza virus was detected in humans, although it caused no serious illness.[45] And in 2003, an H7N7 strain severely affected poultry in the Netherlands, also infecting eighty-three farm workers with a mild illness and killing a veterinarian.

As this is written, the 2004 H5N1 bird-flu epidemic has resumed. Given its documented spread to humans, the possibility of a human epidemic caused by this avian strain of influenza is a definite possibility. Whatever the outcome of this epidemic, it is clear that influenza viruses are undergoing rapid changes, at least partly in response to changing poultry-raising practices. As noted in an editorial in the *Lancet* medical journal: "Live-poultry markets in Asian countries are a breeding ground for avian influenza."[46] In our efforts to streamline farming practices to produce more meat for more people, we have inadvertently created conditions by which a harmless parasite of wild ducks can be converted into a lethal killer of humans.

Should Americans be concerned about this threat? Bird flu has existed for many years in the United States and Canada; in fact, at the same time the H5N1 bird flu epidemic was spreading throughout Southeast Asia, H7 strains of influenza not thought to be pathogenic for humans were infecting chickens in Delaware, Pennsylvania, Texas, and British Columbia.[47] A few poultry workers were infected with the H7 strains, causing mild avian influenza; of greater concern was the diagnosis of H7 avian influenza in a man near New York City who had had no known contact with poultry.[48]

In addition to bird flu's presence in the United States, we have created conditions that may promote the spread of microbes among birds. Poultry farms house as many as eighty thousand chickens, and live-poultry markets can be found in all large cities. According to one expert: "In New York the number of live-poultry markets nearly doubled from 44 in 1994 to over 80 in 2002."[49]

We also import many birds into the United States. By one account: "People who have seen the animal holding facilities at London-Heathrow, New York-Kennedy, and Amsterdam-Schiphol [airports] describe warehouses in which every type of bird and other exotic animal are kept cheek by jowl in conditions resembling those in Guangdong [China] food markets, awaiting trans-shipment. There, poultry can come into close contact with wild-caught birds."[50] For an influenza virus or other microbe that wants to get ahead in life and expand its territory, such conditions are ideal.

10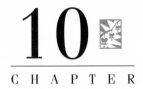

CHAPTER

The Coming Plagues

Lessons from AIDS, West Nile Virus, and Lyme Disease

> *It is therefore as an animal that we must first consider man in his struggles with the environment. For man evolved as an animal, even while he was dreaming of God and the stars.*
>
> RENE DUBOS, *Mirage of Health*, 1959

IN 1969, the bar of human hubris was raised significantly when William H. Stewart, surgeon general of the United States, announced: "The war against infectious diseases has been won."[1] Considering that bacteria, viruses, and protozoa had a more than two-billion-year head start in this war, a victory by recently arrived *Homo sapiens* would be remarkable. In fact, the war against infectious diseases has just begun and is guaranteed to continue for as long as humans inhabit the planet.

Previews of possible future skirmishes against animal microbes occur every day in hundreds of places around the world. We remain unaware of most of these, but a few come to our attention. For example, animal disease outbreaks that occurred in a random two-month period, May and June 2003, and that were reported by ProMED-mail, an Internet service that monitors emerging infectious diseases, included the following:

- A "mystery venereal disease" was affecting baboons in Tanzania, destroying their reproductive organs and causing them to die "in excruciating pain."
- Akabane virus, spread by flying insects, was affecting pregnant cows in Australia, producing "horribly deformed calves which rarely survive."

- Large numbers of monkeys were dying from Kyasanur Forest Disease virus in India, with the outbreak labeled "the most serious in years."
- A case of malignant catarrhal fever, caused by a herpesvirus, was reported among cows, sheep, and pigs in Finland, with an "extremely high mortality" rate.
- The cause of a "mysterious trout disease" in India, identified as an iridovirus, was said to be killing "thousands of trout fish" by causing them to bleed to death.
- An outbreak of gastroenteritis caused by a coronavirus was reported among young pigs in Cuba, with a 43 percent mortality rate.
- An outbreak of bluetongue virus disease was reported among sheep and goats in Brazil.
- A previously unknown disease, probably viral in origin, was spreading among caged parakeets in England and was said to have "a very high death rate."
- African swine fever was reported from the Congo Democratic Republic with "a high mortality rate" among the infected pigs.
- A "highly pathogenic" avian influenza (bird flu) epidemic was being brought under control in the Netherlands, Belgium, and Germany by killing 1.5 million chickens, ducks, and other birds in the affected areas.[2]

Fortunately, most animal disease outbreaks, like those just cited, are caused by microbes that are species specific and therefore do not affect humans. Occasionally, however, when conditions are propitious, animal microbes do cross from one animal species to another. When the new species happens to be humans, the result can be disastrous.

The conditions under which animal microbes are most likely to cross to the human species include changes in human behavior, changes in technology, and changes in ecology.

Human Behavior and AIDS

The microbes that cause human AIDS are primate retroviruses that have existed in African monkeys for millions of years, causing little or no illness in most of them. HIV-2, which causes the milder form of AIDS, is a slight modification of a simian immunodeficiency virus (SIV) carried by sooty mangabey monkeys in West Africa. HIV-1, the more severe form, is a combination of SIV strains carried by two species of monkeys in central Africa. The two strains simultaneously infected a chimpanzee species, *Pan troglodytes troglodytes* and combined into a new strain of SIV, which was then transmitted to humans.[3]

Evidence that supports primates as the source of human HIV is strong. At a molecular level, HIV-1 and HIV-2 are very similar to the viruses carried by the primates. Furthermore, there is an impressive geographic overlap in Central and West Africa where these primates live and where AIDS cases were first seen. Other retroviruses have also been transmitted from primates to humans. For example, simian foamy viruses have been transmitted to humans from chimpanzees, baboons, green monkeys, and macaques.[4] The primate T-cell lymphotropic virus (PTLV-1), another primate retrovirus, was also transmitted from primates to humans; the descendants of these viruses, HTLV-1 and HTLV-2, are important causes of neurological diseases in modern humans.[5] Such cross-species transmission should not surprise us, since primates in general, and chimpanzees in particular, are genetically closely related to humans. As Jared Diamond noted, "the chimpanzees' closest relative is not the gorilla but humans."[6]

Humans in Africa have presumably hunted monkeys and chimpanzees as sources of "bushmeat" for thousands of years. The transmission of SIV from primates to humans could have taken place by a monkey bite, by the virus entering an open sore on human hands that were butchering the animals, or by humans eating undercooked or uncooked primate meat. Such primate-to-human transmission could have taken place multiple times over the years, and, in fact, there is evidence that at least eight independent transmissions did occur.[7]

If transmission of the primate virus to humans took place multiple times in the past, why did AIDS become an epidemic only in the latter years of the twentieth century? The answer to this question is not completely clear but involves several factors, the most important of which are changes in human behavior. AIDS is fundamentally a blood-borne and sexually transmitted disease. Like other sexually transmitted diseases, its pattern of transmission changes as human sexual practices change.

In the 1960s, colonial rule was ending in Africa and there was an outbreak of civil wars. Increased urbanization was followed by social breakdown and widespread prostitution. The African social breakdown was mirrored in developed nations by a sexual revolution in general and a gay revolution in particular, as well as by increased IV drug use and needle sharing. Indeed, if one set out to create the social circumstances most favorable for spreading a sexually transmitted microbe from Africa to the rest of the world, the circumstances in the latter years of the twentieth century would provide a perfect model.

The AIDS epidemic that has resulted from the transmission of primate viruses to humans has been compared to the Black Plague and other great epidemics in history. Since 1980, throughout the world, more than twenty million people have died. Forty million more are already HIV infected; of these, three million were predicted to die in 2003 and the remainder within the next decade. According to a 2002 report, "each day, 14,000 people — 12,000 adults and 2,000 children — become infected with HIV; . . . there will be 45 million new HIV infections by 2010." Sub-Saharan Africa has been most severely affected: In Botswana, 39 percent of the country's adults are infected, and in some sub-Saharan countries, "15 percent or more" of children have been orphaned as AIDS has killed their parents.[8] In the United States, "40,907 new AIDS cases were diagnosed in 1999 and an estimated 41,113 in 2000"; as of mid-2004, an estimated 900,000 Americans were infected with HIV.[9]

The AIDS epidemic, then, illustrates that the transmission of an animal microbe to humans is merely the first step in an epidemic. Many factors played a role in the spread of the disease, including intravenous drug use, its rapid distribution by air travel, and mutations of the virus, but the primary factors that allowed AIDS to become a worldwide epidemic were changes in sexual practices, both locally and internationally.

Technological Changes and West Nile Virus

In August 1999, a physician in Queens, New York, reported to health authorities two cases of individuals with unusual encephalitis-like neurologic symptoms. Within the next week, six more cases had been identified. After interviews of the affected individuals, "the only thing that linked the patients in time and place was that they all had spent time outdoors in their backyards or neighborhoods, especially in the evening hours."[10] This suggested an infectious disease, probably carried by mosquitoes.

The cause of the encephalitis outbreak was ascertained to be the West Nile virus, which had never been seen in the United States. This virus had first been described in Uganda in 1937, near the western branch of the origin of the Nile River. It had caused human encephalitis in Africa, Asia, the Middle East, and Europe but not previously in North America. In recent years, it had caused severe epidemics in Russia, Romania, and Israel. The virus isolated in New York was, in fact, found to be virtually identical to one that had been isolated from the epidemic in Israel.[11]

The West Nile virus is essentially a disease of birds, with mosquitoes used as vectors, and humans as accidental hosts. In two-thirds of humans, it causes no symptoms, but in the other third, it causes fever and occasionally inflammation of the brain (encephalitis). Approximately 7 percent of affected individuals die. Once the virus infects humans, it may also be spread to other humans by blood transfusions.

Although West Nile virus normally spreads by mosquitoes and migrating birds, in 1999 it apparently used an airplane. At least a thousand people travel by air from Israel to New York every day, and it thus seems likely that the virus was brought on a flight to New York either by an infected person or by mosquitoes.[12]

Once in the United States, the virus spread rapidly. In 2001, 66 human cases were recorded in ten states; by 2002, there were 4,161 cases in thirty-seven states, including 284 deaths.[13] An infected dead crow was even found on the grounds of the White House, a reminder that nobody is immune.[14] How much of the rapid spread of West Nile virus is attributable to migrating birds and how much to human-incubating cases carried by airplanes is unclear.

The importance of air travel in disseminating animal microbes is also illustrated by the spread of SARS. On February 21, 2003, a man with SARS stayed overnight at a hotel in Hong Kong, infecting at least seventeen other hotel guests and visitors. Some of the guests, as they were developing SARS, then flew to Hanoi, Singapore, and Toronto, spreading SARS to individuals in those three cities. Still others who had been at the hotel developed SARS and were hospitalized in Hong Kong. A man who visited his sick brother in the Hong Kong hospital then boarded a flight for Beijing and on the flight infected twenty-two other individuals, five of whom died. Retrospective analysis of the seating of passengers on the Beijing flight showed that those sitting immediately in front of, or to the side of, the infected passenger were the most likely to have become infected, presumably through the dissemination of viral particles when the man coughed.[15]

The availability of international air travel has markedly increased the speed at which microbes can spread. Until the middle of the twentieth century, human travel was slower; travelers often developed whatever diseases they might be carrying before they reached their destinations. By contrast, in 2002, there were 532 million passengers on international flights worldwide, including many individuals who took multiple flights.[16] Increasingly, these flights include exotic destinations, so that travelers from Chicago or Copenhagen often return from their exotic vacations carrying exotic microbes.

In addition to human travel, "increasingly, companion animals are accompanying their owners on long-distance travel." This has been facilitated by the recent introduction of a "pet passport scheme" and a loosening of pet-quarantine regulations in many countries.[17] In England, for example, the number of dogs and cats entering the country more than tripled between 2000 and 2003, from 15,871 to 54,572. Not surprisingly, the School of Tropical Medicine in Liverpool reported that cases of "animal diseases picked up on holiday" doubled between 2002 and 2004.[18] Now, not only can humans quickly transport exotic microbes home, but Fido and Fluffy can do so as well.

Air travel is merely one form of modern technology that promotes the spread of microbes, including microbes that have been transmitted from animals to humans. Another technological advance is the widespread availability of syringes. Glass syringes were invented in 1848 but were little used until insulin was introduced in the 1930s. With the availability of penicillin and the invention of inexpensive plastic syringes after World War II, injections became widely used throughout the world. In developed countries, disposable plastic syringes are normally used once and discarded. In developing countries, however, it is common practice to use disposable syringes multiple times without sterilization. Studies have shown that in many countries at least 50 percent of all injections are given with multiple-use, unsterile syringes; in some countries, the figures is as high as 90 percent.[19] It is widely believed by lay persons that injections are more efficacious than medicine given by mouth; injections are therefore big business, and in developing nations they are frequently given by untrained "injection doctors," "needlemen," and a variety of traditional healers.[20]

The widespread use of injections, which can transmit blood-borne microbes from person to person, is a new phenomenon. Since hominids evolved six million years ago, the only routes open for most microbes to breach human defenses have been through the mouth, intestine, respiratory system, genital tract, and open wounds. Injecting microbes directly into the muscles and bloodstream of humans is analogous to opening the gates of a city under siege. The World Health Organization estimates that, worldwide, twelve *billion* syringes are sold each year for injections, sufficient for two injections for every man, woman, and child if each syringe is used only once. Studies have estimated that in some countries in Southeast Asia and the eastern Mediterranean regions, where syringes are often used multiple times, each man, woman, and child receives an average of three unsterile injections each year.[21] The use of unsterile syringes is thought to have played a role in spreading the AIDS virus, as well as hepatitis B and C, malaria, Ebola virus, and Lassa fever.[22]

Another technological advance that threatens to increase the transmission of animal microbes to humans is xenotransplantation, the transplanting of animal organs into humans. The procedure was first carried out in 1910, when a monkey kidney was transplanted into a young girl suffering from renal failure. In 1963, kidneys from chimpanzees were put into six patients with renal failure, but the longest any patient lived was nine months.[23] Since that time, primates have been largely ruled out as sources for human organs, both because of ethical concerns and because of the danger of transmitting primate microbes to humans.[24]

In recent years, there has been increasing interest in transplanting pig organs and tissues to humans. Experiments are underway using pig hearts for patients with heart failure, pig nerve cells for patients with Huntington's disease or Parkinson's disease, and pig pancreatic cells for patients with diabetes. Commercial interest is strong, with projections that xenotransplants could become a $6 billion market by 2010.[25]

The need for a supply of human organs is acute. At any given time, more than fifty thousand individuals are on organ waiting lists, and most will die before human organs become available. In addition to their limited availability, transplanted human organs can transmit microbes such as hepatitis C and cytomegalovirus. The limited availability and danger of using human organs for transplantation must be weighed against the dangers of using animals' organs. Pigs, like all animals, carry a variety of infectious agents, including a hepatitis virus, at least three herpesviruses, a paramyxovirus, a torovirus, and a circovirus, although to date the evidence for transmission of these viruses to humans is scant.[26] Of greatest concern is an endogenous retrovirus carried by pigs that is integrated into the genome and can infect human cells.[27] Many of these viruses cause no problems in pigs but could be pathogenic if transplanted into humans. If xenotransplantation becomes widespread, therefore, it will provide a new route for microbes to move from animals to humans.

Bioterrorism will also be affected by technology and thereby increase human exposure to animal microbes. These include microbes such as smallpox, anthrax, brucellosis, Q fever, tularemia, and glanders, which have been known for thousands of years, as well as microbes that have apparently moved from animals to humans more recently, such as Ebola virus and Lassa virus.[28] Technologically sophisticated bioterrorists are likely to discover new methods for unleashing these microbes. Even more worrisome are potential uses of the growing field of synthetic biology to modify existing microbes so that, for example, they could be used to neutralize the human body's existing defenses or negate the effect of anti-infective medications.[29] With bioterrorism come wars, which promote the spread of microbes through unsanitary living conditions and malnutrition. As Hans Zinsser noted: "Soldiers have rarely won wars. They more often mop up after the barrage of epidemics. . . . The epidemics get the blame for defeat, the generals get the credit for victory. It ought to be the other way around."[30]

Ecological Changes and Lyme Disease

In October 1999, the Institute of Medicine held a workshop on emerging infectious diseases. Ecological changes, including urbanization, global warming, and changes in forestation, were among the more prominent factors cited as contributing to the spread of microbes.[31]

It is not generally appreciated that big cities are a relatively recent phenomenon. For the first eight thousand years after humans settled into villages, the population of the largest settlements rarely exceeded 20,000 inhabitants. By 1000 B.C.E., only four cities in the world had populations of 50,000 or more. In the fourteenth century, Paris, with 100,000 people, was the largest city in Europe, and as late as 1840, New York was the largest city in the United States, with 250,000 inhabitants.

Megacities, with populations of ten million or more, are new. New York in 1950 was the first to surpass that mark, but by 2000, fourteen other cities in the world had joined it. In 2015, there are projected to be twenty-one megacities, five of which (Bombay, Delhi, Dhaka, Tokyo, and Sao Paulo) are expected to have populations of more than twenty million.[32] Such population concentrations are likely to create novel patterns of infectious disease transmission and also lead to the emergence of new microbes that require huge populations for their natural reservoirs. Urbanization also promotes the spread of microbes through contaminated water supplies, poor sewage systems, trash heaps that attract rodents, and crowded living conditions. As noted in 1998 by one expert on emerging infections: "The mega cities of the tropics, with their lack of sanitary systems, serve as incubators for emerging zoonoses—they represent the most difficult zoonotic diseases risks of the next century."[33]

Global warming has been widely discussed as a phenomenon likely to increase the distribution of infectious diseases. It is projected, for example, that global warming could lead to the reemergence in such cities as New York, Rome, and Tokyo of the protozoa and viruses that cause malaria, yellow fever, and dengue.[34] Other infectious diseases whose spread would be favored by a rise in temperature include viral encephalitis, schistosomiasis, and leishmaniasis.[35]

Deforestation, reforestation, irrigation, dam building, and alterations in agriculture can also bring about ecological change. All have been known to produce changes in the transmission of microbes. Argentine hemorrhagic fever, for example, increased sharply among humans in South America following the conversion of grasslands to maize cultivation, a change that favored the rodent, the natural reservoir for the virus that causes this disease.[36]

The best example in the United States of a rise in a human disease brought about by ecological change that affects an animal microbe is Lyme disease. The disease is caused by a spirochetal bacteria, *Borrelia burgdoferi*, that is transmitted to humans by ticks. Ticks have a complex life cycle, taking two years to mature and then attaching themselves to mammals such as deer, which have become the main natural reservoir for Lyme disease.

Deer were plentiful in the eastern United States when Europeans first colonized it. As forests were turned into fields and deer were killed for their meat, deer became rare. In 1854, for example, when Henry David Thoreau wrote *Walden*, he said that deer had not been seen in his part of Massachusetts for eighty years.[37]

After the Civil War, many New Englanders moved westward to more fertile land, allowing their fields to return to woodland. By 1980, northeastern states had four times more forested area than they had in 1860, and this trend has continued as more farms have been abandoned. In contrast to the forests of the early nineteenth century, however, the reforested areas have almost no cougars, wolves, bears, or other predators that previously kept the deer population in check.

In the early twentieth century, deer returned to the reforested areas, now devoid of natural predators. They multiplied steadily until, in the last two decades, their population exploded. There are now thought to be at least as many deer in the United States as there were when the colonists arrived, but the deer are concentrated in smaller, often suburban, areas. As one study concluded, deer "are now as commonly noted as squirrels in some suburban communities."[38]

One measure of deer population is how often they are hit by vehicles. According to a recent U.S. survey, deer "are struck by cars, trucks, and motorcycles more than a million times a year, with the accidents killing more than 100 people annually. . . . The human toll makes deer deadlier than sharks, alligators, bears, and rattlesnakes combined." In Connecticut, between 1995 and 2000, "the number of drivers who reported hitting a deer rose 297 percent." In addition, according to the Federal Aviation Administration, at airports "deer have been struck by more than 500 aircraft over the last decade, including fighter jets and Boeing 737's."[39]

While deer were moving into suburban woodlands, people were moving out of cities and building houses next to the woodlands. The homeowners proceeded to plant their lawns with flowers, vegetables, and shrubs that deer like to eat. The suburbanites brought along their dogs and cats, which can also be affected by Lyme disease and can bring ticks from the adjoining woods into the house, thus making it easier for them to infect humans.

The current epidemic of Lyme disease in the United States is a natural and predictable consequence of the exploding deer population. Since the initial 1977 outbreak in Lyme, Connecticut, the incidence of the disease has risen sharply. In the decade between 1991 and 2000, the number of newly affected individuals doubled to almost eighteen thousand per year, even as cases continued to be underreported.[40] In 2002, reported cases of Lyme disease increased to 23,763 and are apparently continuing to increase. Children are most commonly affected, but individuals of all ages are vulnerable. The initial signs, flulike symptoms and a rash, if untreated, may be followed by arthritis and complications of the central nervous system or heart, including meningitis, encephalitis, paralysis of the facial nerves, psychiatric symptoms, or heart-rhythm abnormalities.[41] Untreated, Lyme disease may become a chronic and disabling illness that continues for many years.

The Great Unknown

The greatest danger in the transmission of microbes from animals to humans is not what we know but what we don't know. As noted in chapter 1, researchers compiled a list of 1,415 microbes known to cause diseases in humans.[42] One can compare that number to the estimated three hundred thousand to one million different species of bacteria and the five thousand species of viruses thought to exist, the vast majority of which have not yet been identified.

We should also remember that humans are merely one of 4,500 species of mammals and that almost all research on microbes has been done on those that are presently thought to affect humans. Except for laboratory rodents, which have been studied for research purposes, we know almost nothing about microbes that infect other mammals, to say nothing of microbes that infect birds, reptiles, amphibians, fish, or simpler forms of life. In short, we are aware of only a tiny fraction of microbes that may cause disease in humans; we should therefore be very modest about our ability to predict the microbial effects of any changes in the relationship between humans and other animals.

As molecular studies proceed, it is inevitable that additional human diseases will be identified as caused by animal microbes. Of particular interest is the role of microbes in chronic human diseases, since the identification of these relationships requires the application of sophisticated molecular techniques that are just starting to be applied to the study of chronic diseases. What, for example, is the relationship between *Chlamydia pneumonia* and human coronary disease? This microbe has been found in coronary artery plaques in many people with this disease.[43] The human strain of *Chlamydia pneumonia* appears to be closely related to the strain found in horses, which could conceivably have been the origin of this pathogen before it became adapted to human-to-human transmission.[44]

The possible relationship of human cancers to animal cancers is another area that is mostly unknown. Cancer is a leading cause of death in dogs; cancer of the breast, testes, and bone are especially common.[45] Cats are especially affected by leukemias and lymphomas. Experimental work has shown that some human microbes may cause cancer when injected into animals.[46] And some human cancers, such as cancer of the stomach, liver, and cervix, have been linked to microbes such as *Helicobacter pylori*, hepatitis B virus, and human papilloma viruses, respectively. Whether or not any human cancers will ultimately be associated with exposure to animals remains to be determined, but anecdotal accounts of humans and their pets being diagnosed with similar cancers are intriguing.[47]

What Can Be Done?

Viewed in historical perspective, human health has improved significantly in recent centuries. The world's population has increased from 2 billion in 1875 to 6.3 billion today. Those with access to modern medicine and antibiotics have a quality of life much better than that of their forebears.

At the same time, as noted by infectious disease specialists, the "emergence of new zoonotic pathogens seems to be increasing."[48] The recent emergence of AIDS, SARS, monkeypox, West Nile virus, bird flu, and other infections, all caused by microbes transmitted from animals to humans, should be regarded as a wake-up call. In 2003, the Institute of Medicine published a report from its Committee on Emerging Microbial Threats to Health in the Twenty-first Century. The tone of the report was sober and subdued: "As the work of this Committee draws to an end, none of its members are sanguine about what the future may hold with respect to microbial threats to health. . . . Today's outlook with regard to microbial threats is bleak on a number of fronts. . . . Microbial threats present us with new surprises every year.[49]

The most urgent task, according to the report, is "to strengthen global infectious disease surveillance . . . to recognize previously unknown illnesses or unusual outbreaks of disease that may have global significance."[50] Currently, one effective network set up to accomplish this task is the Program for Monitoring Emerging Diseases, or ProMED, an Internet reporting system administered by the International Society for Infectious Diseases using foundation funding. Similarly, the World Health Organization (WHO) launched the Global Outbreak Alert and Response Network in 2000 but, like many WHO endeavors, it has been slow to reach its potential because of the politics of that organization.

A fundamental problem at both international and national levels is a lack of coordination between agencies that have responsibility for animal health and agencies that have responsibility for human health. Internationally, the World Organization for Animal Health (Office International des Epizooties, OIE), based in Paris, has responsibility for animal diseases, whereas the World Health Organization, based in Geneva, has responsibility for human diseases. Coordination between these two separate agencies has traditionally been very poor. Influenza for example, is a disease of great importance for both poultry and humans. According to the 2003 Institute of Medicine report, OIE is interested in "only certain influenza virus types that are highly pathogenic for poultry, . . . those viruses that are found to be rather nonpathogenic in poultry, but for which a potential threat to humans exists, are ignored." [51]

At the national level, cooperation between agencies responsible for animal and human health has been equally deficient. In the United States, for example, the Department of Defense (DOD) operates infectious disease research laboratories in five countries (Egypt, Indonesia, Kenya, Peru, and Thailand). DOD also collects infectious disease information at the Armed Forces Intelligence Center and through an Electronic Surveillance System for Early Notification of Community-Based Epidemics (ESSENCE) at military facilities worldwide. The Centers for Disease Control and Prevention (CDC) collects data from states on notifiable infectious diseases and publishes them weekly in *Morbidity and Mortality Weekly Reports*. These data include, however, only selected and recognized diseases. In response to the threats of bioterrorism, CDC recently also launched a National Electronic Disease Surveillance System (NEDSS) and a Web-based communications network for public health officials (Epi-X).

Yet information on animal diseases in the United States is not the responsibility of either DOD or CDC, but of the Animal and Plant Health Inspection Service (APHIS) of the Department of Agriculture. APHIS employs more than three hundred U.S. and host-country nationals in twenty-seven countries, with the primary mission of protecting U.S. animal and plant resources from agricultural pests and diseases, such as foot-and-mouth disease; thus, its focus is on protecting animals and plants, not people. APHIS also operates a laboratory at Plum Island, off the coast of Long Island, which is the major U.S. facility for research on animal microbes from foreign countries.

These various government agencies are poorly coordinated, despite some of them, like CDC, individually doing excellent work. In 1992, the Institute of Medicine, in its report *Emerging Infections*, noted that "there is little coordination among these [federal] agencies and organizations regarding infectious diseases surveillance." [52] Ten years later, another Institute of Medicine report described "evidence of new turf tensions" between the federal agencies: "The risk that this will get worse affects zoonotic disease episodes in particular, where laboratory and field activities resemble research projects and many different specialists must be involved. In several recent zoonotic episodes, however, scientists became competitive and insular, seeming to worry more about their publications than about the public's health." [53]

Federal agencies with responsibility for different aspects of West Nile virus, for example, are these:

- Centers for Disease Control and Prevention (CDC): Reporting and investigation of human cases

- Food and Drug Administration (FDA): Protection of blood supply against contamination by the virus
- National Institutes of Health (NIH): Research on the virus
- Department of Defense (DOD): Research on the virus
- Department of Agriculture: Surveillance and reporting of the effect of the virus on poultry and livestock
- Department of the Interior: Assistance to states with diagnosis of the virus among birds and other wildlife
- Department of Commerce: Research on mosquito populations; plans for controlling mosquitoes
- Environmental Protection Agency: Research on pesticides used in prevention efforts[54]

The lack of federal agency coordination is especially evident for microbes that are transmitted from animals to humans, such as West Nile virus, SARS, BSE, and monkeypox. In mid-2004, several members of Congress publicly urged Tommy Thompson, secretary of the Department of Health and Human Services, to create a task force to coordinate research on diseases such as BSE.[55] Until this lack is remedied, Americans will remain unnecessarily vulnerable to animal-transmitted diseases. One of the major recommendations of the 2003 Institute of Medicine report, in fact, was that "the overseas diseases surveillance activities of the relevant U.S. agencies . . . should be coordinated by a single federal agency, such as CDC."[56]

A basic cause of this lack of coordination of disease information is a gulf that has long existed between veterinarians, the specialists in animal diseases, and infectious disease physicians, the specialists in human diseases. The two groups have trained in different schools and have worked in different professional worlds for more than a century. Although it has become increasingly clear that most emerging human infectious diseases originate in animals, little effort has been made to bridge this gulf. The lack of coordination between animal- and human-disease specialists was highlighted again during the recent bird-flu epidemic. "Medical and veterinary schools need to cooperate more," noted Frederick Murphy, an expert on zoonoses.[57] A model for such coordination exists in Denmark, which has developed "a zoonosis center as an element of its national public health institution, . . . uniting veterinary and human health professionals."[58]

Another aspect of disease surveillance that needs improvement is the autopsy rate. In 1964, 41 percent of all persons who died in U.S. hospitals underwent autopsy, which is useful to pinpoint the cause of death and to detect new diseases as they emerge. Since 1964, the autopsy rate in U.S. hospitals has fallen progressively; it is now only 5 percent.[59] By not doing more autopsies, especially ones that use sophisticated molecular techniques to identify microbes, we are missing one of our best opportunities to detect emerging microbes and diseases that may be transmitted from animals to humans.

Coordinating veterinary and medical personnel in a single center would also be very useful for advancing research on microbes being transmitted from animals to humans. The CDC, the Department of Defense, and the National Institute of Allergy and Infectious Disease (NIAID) under NIH are all carrying out important research on infectious diseases, but research on animal diseases is the responsibility of the Department of Agriculture. Given what is now known about the importance of zoonoses, it is illogical to have research on bird flu in poultry carried out by one government agency and research on bird flu in humans carried out by another.

For reducing exposure to animal microbes at an individual level, each of us must decide how much and what kind of contact we want to have with pet animals, and parents must make this decision for their children. It is possible to keep a pet and minimize exposure to animal-transmitted microbes by choosing a nonexotic pet and by following commonsense principles, the most important of which are related to hand washing after pet contact, observing other aspects of personal hygiene, and ensuring that pet immunizations are up to date. Individuals may wish to keep exotic animals as pets, but this falls into the category of high-risk behavior, along with motorcycle riding and skydiving, and the risk to other family members must also be taken into consideration. Another important principle for minimizing one's exposure to animal microbes is to cook eggs, meat, and other food to recommended temperatures to reduce transmission opportunities for food-borne microbes.

It is clear, however, that regulations need to be revisited for the importation of exotic animals. Currently, dogs imported into the United States must have been vaccinated against rabies at least thirty days before importation, and dogs and cats must undergo quarantine in some states. For exotic animals, however, there are few restrictions. The Department of Agriculture Web site states explicitly: "We do not have any regulations or restrictions on the importation of fish, reptiles, lions, tigers, bears, foxes, monkeys, endangered species, guinea pigs, hamsters, gerbils, mice, rats, chinchillas, squirrels, mongoose, chipmunks, ferrets, or other rodents provided they have not been inoculated with any pathogens for scientific purposes."[60] It is not just a question of whether these animals have been inoculated with pathogens; it is also a question of what pathogens they are already carrying.

Perhaps the most important activity for minimizing the transmission of microbes from animals to humans is education. Most people are unaware of the potential of animals to cause human disease. In one study, for example, only two out of thirty-two dog owners "expressed awareness that diseases other than rabies could be transmitted from pet dogs to human beings."[61] Another survey regarding "pet-associated health risks" reported that "pediatricians' knowledge was incomplete, parents' knowledge even more so, and anticipatory guidance about pets notably lacking." Still another survey found that "most physicians felt uncomfortable advising patients about the health risks of animal contact and indicated that veterinarians should play a greater role."[62]

Owners of pet stores also have a responsibility to educate customers. One study examined the role of pet-store managers in advising individuals who buy animals regarding their possible disease transmission to humans. It was found that "only 23 percent of owners/managers of pet shops advised customers of the potential zoonotic risks from puppies." Giving medicine to puppies to kill the dog's intestinal worms is widely recommended as standard procedure, but in this survey, "four petshops advised customers to worm themselves and/or their children as preventive measures for parasitic infection of their dogs."[63]

In summary, the relationship between humans and other animals is marked by contradictions. Domesticated animals have provided us with food, clothing, and other essentials, making our civilization possible. At the same time, animals have transmitted to humans microbes that have caused, and are causing, many of our worst diseases. At a personal level, we regard ourselves as far superior to other members of Phylum Craniata, Subphyulum Vertebrata, Class Mammalia — the beasts of the earth — and yet we treat these other animals, when they are our pets, as if they are one of us.

It seems certain that we will experience additional epidemics of human diseases that will be transmitted to us from animals. Popular representations of such epidemics depict them as arising in the jungles of Africa or the rainforests of South America. Ebola, Lassa, Marburg, Machupo — these are the dreaded and deadly "andromeda strains" that Hollywood portrays and about which we worry. In fact, the coming human plagues are equally likely to come from an exotic pet kinkajou in New York, a pet prairie dog in Chicago, or even a child's kitten in Los Angeles. It is not a question of *whether* we will experience such plagues, but rather a question of *when* and *how often*.

11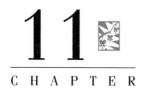

CHAPTER

A Four-Footed View of History

That men do not learn very much from the lessons of history is the most important of all the lessons that history has to teach.

ALDOUS HUXLEY

*H*OMO *sapiens* has had a peculiar history. For almost a million years, we wandered the world as hunters, living in small groups but creating no permanent civilizations. Then, approximately ten thousand years ago, we domesticated plants and animals; in the following eight thousand years, we created city-states, monuments, centralized governments, art, architecture, literature, and philosophy. Thus, during less than 1 percent of our time as a species, we went from being peripatetic nomads to the likes of Aristotle and Cicero.

The remains of these early civilizations—the pyramids of Egypt, sculptures of Greece, and temples of Rome—are indeed impressive. The Harrapan cities in the Indus Valley five thousand years ago had elaborate sewage systems that one can still see in ruins such as Mohenjo Daro. Roman cities more than two thousand years ago had aqueducts to bring water, public baths that accommodated hundreds of people, and public lavatories "fitted with marble urinals, . . . a small charge being made for admission." The first public lavatories in London did not open until 1851. It has been said that "in its cleanliness, sanitation and water supply, Rome was much more akin to twentieth-century London and New York than to medieval Paris or eighteenth-century Vienna."[1]

Domesticated animals played a large role in these evolving civilizations. For example, at Tell Leilan, which increased in size sixfold between 2600 and 2400 B.C.E. as a political center for northern Mesopotamia, the inhabitants kept pigs, sheep, goats, and cattle, and used horses and mules for transportation.[2] The shards, paintings, friezes, and other relics of these early civilizations clearly illustrate the importance of domesticated animals—Sumerian sheep and pigs, Persian horses and water buffalo, Chinese ducks and geese, Egyptian cattle and cats, Minoan bulls and goats, Roman hunting dogs and chickens.

It seems reasonable to conclude that without domesticated animals to provide meat, clothing, and transportation and to guard the sheep and grain, these early civilizations would not have evolved.

Equally as impressive as the rise of these civilizations was their fall. In Mesopotamia in approximately 2200 B.C.E., there occurred a "sudden collapse of the Akkadian empire." Excavations at Tell Leilan have shown that it was "suddenly abandoned" and that "similar abandonments are evident at almost all excavated sites of this period across the Habur and Assyrian Plains."[3] Most of the ancient civilizations did not decline as precipitously as the Akkadian Empire did, but a pattern of decline can be traced in all of them: Civilizations grew and flourished for hundreds of years, then withered for a period and eventually died.

Historians have speculated exhaustively on reasons why ancient civilizations fell. Drought and other climatic changes are certainly part of the answer. This has been cited as the main reason for the sudden demise of the Akkadian Empire,[4] and similar climatic changes affected Egypt, the Indus River Valley, and the Aegean area at this time. Civil unrest and wars, famine, and natural disasters such as floods, earthquakes, volcanic eruptions, and infestations of locusts also played a role and often occurred in combination.

Perhaps the most important reason for the decline of ancient civilizations, however, was the spread of infectious diseases, most of which were caused by microbes that had spread to humans from domesticated animals. Measles, smallpox, tuberculosis, bubonic plague, typhus, dysentery, dengue, diphtheria, influenza, yellow fever, malaria, pertussis, polio, cholera, schistosomiasis, and leprosy probably all existed as human diseases by the sixth century C.E., when the last of the ancient civilizations, the Roman Empire, finally expired.

Fragmentary evidence supports the important role played by infectious diseases. For example, in 480 B.C.E., when Xerxes attempted to expand his Persian Empire by invading Greece, dysentery struck his army, reducing it by more than a third. As R. S. Bray notes in *Armies of Pestilence*, dysentery was "the final nail in the coffin of the Persian pretensions in Greece and the Mediterranean world. . . . It might be claimed with justification that Greek and European culture owe their continued existence to Greek arms and dysentery." The defeat threw the Persian Empire "into a state of languid torpor, from which it could not rise again."[5]

Fifty years later, in 430 B.C.E., Athenian civilization was at its zenith and also at war with Sparta. A severe disease, never definitively identified, struck Athens and its fleet, killing at least one-third of the population, including Pericles and many other political and military leaders. As described by Thucydides, those afflicted suffered from coughing, vomiting, diarrhea, and terrible skin sores. "Unable to bear the touch of clothes or bedding, they staggered naked through the streets. . . . They died in streets, in temples, in wells into which they had fallen." Thucydides, who himself was afflicted, noted: "Words indeed fail when one tries to give a general picture of this disease; and as for the suffering of individuals, they seemed almost beyond the capacity of human nature to endure."[6]

The Athenian epidemic was followed by widespread tuberculosis, described by Hippocrates in 400 B.C.E. The diseases led to the eventual defeat of Athens and its demise as a major power. According to Arno Karlen's *Man and Microbes*, "Athens would never fully regain its political and cultural glory. More than 2,000 years later the West's finest minds would still dream of recreating the golden age that the plague had helped destroy."[7]

Egypt also suffered from epidemic diseases that contributed to its downfall. Evidence from Egyptian mummies suggest that smallpox, tuberculosis, malaria, schistosomiasis, and polio all occurred.[8] Old Testament stories describe a "very severe plague" of Egyptian cattle and another epidemic that was characterized by "boils breaking out in sores on man and beast."[9] Still another disease, according to Exodus, killed "all the first-born in the land of Egypt . . . and all the first-born of the cattle."[10] However apocryphal, such stories suggest that epidemic diseases were important events in ancient Egypt.

In the East, the Harrapan civilization flourished in the Indus River Valley from approximately 3000 to 1800 B.C.E. but then rapidly declined. Although warfare and drought played a role, Paul Ewald has proposed that the spread of cholera was also an important factor.[11] In China, "mention of unusual outbreaks of disease abound in the Han dynastic history, . . . including some that acted in epidemic fashion from time to time."[12] Measles and smallpox are both thought to have existed, and "from 200 B.C. to A.D. 200 [China's] population declined severely because of new epidemics."[13] In 310–312 C.E., an epidemic disease, "preceded by locusts and famine, left only one or two out of a hundred persons alive in the northwestern provinces of China; and this was followed ten years later, in 322, by another epidemic in which two or three out of ten died over a wider region of the country."[14] The effect of such epidemic was to bring to a close the Han Empire, which then "fell like a rotten tree before a gale."[15]

It is the Roman Empire, however, for which the most definitive records link infectious diseases to its decline. The historian Livy "records at least eleven cases of pestilential disaster in republican times, the earliest dated 387 B.C."[16] One of the most severe of these was the "plague on Antoninus," which raged from 165 to 180 C.E. It was brought to Rome by soldiers returning from Syria and is estimated to have killed one-quarter to one-third of the Roman population, including Emperor Marcus Aurelius. Some historians have designated this epidemic "the turning point of the Roman Empire," the beginning of its decline.[17]

Even more severe was the plague of Cyprian, which lasted from 250 to 265 C.E. Edward Gibbon claimed that it "raged without interruption in every province, every city, and almost every family of the Roman empire. During some time, five thousand persons died daily in Rome, and many towns . . . were entirely depopulated."[18] The epidemic not only affected the Roman Empire but spread throughout Europe and is said to have killed over half its population: "More died than survived, and not sufficient people were left to bury the dead."[19] According to one source, the plague of Cyprian "indisputably changed the course of history in western Europe."[20]

The precise microbial causes of these Roman epidemics have never been ascertained, although smallpox and measles have been suggested as candidates. However, the cause of the final epidemic to devastate the Roman Empire, the plague of Justinian, has been clearly identified as *Yersina pestis*, the bacteria that causes bubonic plague. As described in chapter 6, this epidemic raged for more than fifty years in the sixth century C.E., initially devastating the eastern Mediterranean and then spreading to Italy, where, according to Gibbon, "the harvest and the vintage withered on the ground."[21] From Italy, it spread from city to city along the Mediterranean coast, carried by infected rats on ships, eventually reaching England. Estimates of the total dead from this plague are as high as 100 million, but the true number is unknown.[22] The plague devastated trade and the economy of the Mediterranean region and altered the course of history. As a consequence of the Justinian plague, it has been speculated that "the relatively plague-free nomads and barbarians moved in to settle or graze the land," "enormous areas . . . became Islamicised," "letters and art in Europe entered the Dark Ages," and "monastic life took a stranglehold on the intellectual mainstream of the Christian world."[23]

According to Hans Zinsser's *Rats, Lice and History*, the Justinian plague was "the coupe de grâce to the ancient empire." Zinsser suggests that "the calamitous epidemics which—sweeping the Roman world again and again during its most turbulent political periods—must have exerted a material, if not decisive, influence upon the final outcome."[24]

We are not arguing that infectious diseases alone caused the decline of ancient civilizations. Natural disasters, famine, and warfare often work in unison with microbes to bring about the final result. Warfare and natural disasters, for example, often destroy farm animals and crops, whose scarcity leads to famines; these in turn weaken people's immune systems, making them more susceptible to infectious diseases. Conversely, infectious diseases, especially in epidemic waves, have secondary consequences: They demoralize populations and undermine human authority. Lawlessness was a common denominator during many of the world's great epidemics. As Zinsser notes: "The effects of a succession of epidemics upon a state are not measurable in mortalities alone. Whenever pestilences have attained particularly terrifying proportions, their secondary consequences have been much more far-reaching and disorganizing than anything that could have resulted from the mere numerical reduction of the population."[25]

Some historians have also suggested that ancient disease epidemics contributed to the rise of Christianity and other world religions. Since the microbial origins of epidemics were unknown, their cause was usually attributed to divine acts. As William McNeil noted in *Plagues and People*, Christianity had an advantage over paganism insofar as "faith made life meaningful even amid sudden and surprising death."[26] The promise of physical resurrection after death and of life everlasting offered great solace during periods when large numbers of people were dying.

Conversions to Christianity were more common during epidemics and natural disasters. This is illustrated impressively by the Roman "plague of Cyprian," which took its name from St. Cyprian, the bishop of Carthage. At its height, Cyprian and his fellow priests "baptized as many as two or three hundred persons a day."[27] He wrote a tract extolling the epidemic:

> Many of us are dying in this mortality, that is many of us are being freed from the world. This mortality is a bane to the Jews and pagans and enemies of Christ; to the servants of God it is a salutary departure. As to the fact that without any discrimination in the human race the just are dying with the unjust, it is not for you to think that the destruction is a common one for both the evil and the good. The just are called to refreshment, the unjust are carried off to torture; protection is more quickly given to the faithful; punishment to the faithless. . . . How suitable, how necessary it is that this plague and pestilence, which seems horrible and deadly, searches out the justice of each and every one and examines the minds of the human race.[28]

Cartwright and Biddiss in *Disease and History* suggest that "Christianity would hardly have succeeded in establishing itself as a world force . . . if the Roman Empire had not been ravaged by incurable disease during the years which followed the life of Christ." Zinsser similarly noted that "Christianity owes a formidable debt to bubonic plague and to smallpox, no less than to earthquake and volcanic eruptions."[29]

In proposing this four-footed view of history, we have necessarily focused on the epidemic diseases, such as smallpox, measles, and bubonic plague, which were so momentous that they were recorded as written history. No less devastating, perhaps, were endemic human diseases also originating in animals. Thus, tuberculosis, dysentery, pertussis, and other diseases almost certainly occurred in small outbreaks, killing farmers who supplied food to the cities along with government leaders, military commanders, artisans, and philosophers. This ongoing loss of population was an important contributor to the decline of ancient civilizations, although it is much less visible because it was not usually passed down in recorded history.

In conclusion, the great civilizations of the ancient world came into existence in the centuries following the domestication of plants and animals. Sheep, goats, pigs, cattle, horses, and other domesticated animals played a major role in making such civilizations possible. At the same time, domesticated animals brought with them their microbes, many of which adapted to humans, causing infectious diseases. As people in ancient civilizations became urbanized and transportation improved, infectious diseases spread more easily, some in epidemic fashion. These diseases played a major role in the decline of these civilizations. The role of animals, therefore, was to be both a cause and a curse, contributing to the creation and then the dissolution of civilizations that, even today, we regard as extraordinary.

Notes

CHAPTER 1. The Smallest Passengers on Noah's Ark

1. L. K. Altman, "Patient May Have Transmitted Monkeypox," *New York Times,* June 13, 2003; "An Ounce Of Prevention: Some Early Lessons and Legacies of SARS," *Economist,* June 7, 2003, 79; ProMED-mail, "West Nile Virus, Human: USA (South Carolina)," June 15, 2003, accessed at http://www.promedmail.org; ProMED-mail, "West Nile Virus Update 2003: USA," June 13, 2003; ProMED-mail, "Hantavirus Pulmonary Syndrome: USA," June 2, 2003; "Notifiable Diseases/Deaths in Selected Cities Weekly Information," *Morbidity and Mortality Weekly Report* 52 (2003): 551–559; D. G. McNeil Jr., "Researchers Have New Theory on Origin of AIDS Virus," *New York Times,* June 13, 2003; S. Blakeslee, "Mad Cows, Sane Cats: Making Sense of the 'Species Barrier,'" *New York Times,* June 3, 2003; R. Stein, "Infections Now More Widespread: Animals Passing Them to Humans," *Washington Post,* June 15, 2003.
2. Lynn Margulis and Karlene V. Schwartz, *Five Kingdoms: An Illustrated Guide to the Phyla of Life on Earth* (New York: W. H. Freeman, 2001), 208.
3. Stephen Jay Gould, Foreword, in Margulis and Schwartz, *Five Kingdoms.*
4. Rita Colwell, quoted in Laurie Garrett, *The Coming Plague* (New York: Penguin, 1994), 561.
5. K. Sawyer, "Oldest Living Bacteria Are Revived," *Washington Post,* October 19, 2000.
6. G. L. Simon and S. L. Gorbach, "Intestinal Flora in Health and Disease," *Gastroenterology* 86 (1984): 174–193; M. N. Swartz, "Human Diseases Caused by Foodborne Pathogens of Animal Origin," *Human Disease and Foodborne Pathogens* 34 (supp. 3) (2002): S111–S122.
7. F. Guarner and J.-R. Malagelada, "Gut Flora in Health and Disease," *Lancet* 360 (2003): 512–519.
8. Tony McMichael, *Human Frontiers, Environments, and Disease* (Cambridge: Cambridge University Press, 2001), 376n11.
9. P. A. Mackowiak, "The Normal Microbial Flora," *New England Journal of Medicine* 307 (1982): 83–93.
10. J. O. Andersson, W. F. Doolittle, and C. L. Nesbø, "Are There Bugs in Our Genome?" *Science* 292 (2001): 1848–1850.
11. Robin Marantz Henig, *A Dancing Matrix: How Science Confronts Emerging Viruses* (New York: Vintage Books, 1994), 76; A. J. Nahmias and D. C. Reanney, "The Evolution of Viruses," *Annual Reviews in Ecology and Systematics* 8 (1977): 29–49.
12. Lewis Thomas, *The Lives of a Cell* (New York: Penguin, 1978), 5.
13. Mark Twain, *Letters from the Earth* (New York: Harper and Row, 1962), letter 7.
14. L. D. Martin, "Earth History, Disease, and the Evolution of Primates," in Charles Greenblatt and Mark Spigelman, eds., *Emerging Pathogens* (New York: Oxford University Press, 2003), 13–24.
15. Hans Zinsser, *Rats, Lice, and History* (1934; repr. Boston: Little, Brown, 1963), 57.

16. Jared Diamond, *Guns, Germs, and Steel* (New York: W. W. Norton, 1999), 209.
17. Arno Karlen, *Man and Microbes: Disease and Plagues in History and Modern Times* (New York: Simon and Schuster, 1996), 16, 18.
18. Paul W. Ewald, "Evolution and Ancient Diseases: the Roles Of Genes, Germs, and Transmission Modes," in Charles Greenblatt and Mark Spigelman, eds., *Emerging Pathogens* (New York: Oxford University Press, 2003), 117–124. For a complete discussion of this topic, see Paul W. Ewald, *Evolution of Infectious Disease* (New York: Oxford University Press, 1994).
19. Richard Fiennes, *Man, Nature, and Disease* (New York: Signet, 1964), 91.
20. M. Höcker and P. Hohenberger, "*Helicobacter pylori* Virulence Factors: One Part of a Big Picture," *Lancet* 362 (2003): 1231–1233.
21. R. Bellamy, C. Ruwende, T. Corrah et al., "Variations in the *NRAMP1* Gene and Susceptibility to Tuberculosis in West Africans," *New England Journal of Medicine* 338 (1998): 640–644; R. J. Wilkinson, M. Llewelyn, Z. Toossi et al., "Influence of Vitamin D Deficiency and Vitamin D Receptor Polymorphisms on Tuberculosis among Gujarati Asians in West London: A Case-Control Study," *Lancet* 355 (2000): 618–621.
22. E. Pennisi, "Close Encounters: Good, Bad, and Ugly," *Science* 290 (2000): 1491–1493.
23. Fiennes, *Man, Nature and Disease*, 88.
24. W. Plowright, "The Effects of Rinderpest and Rinderpest Control on Wildlife in Africa," *Symposia of the Zoological Society of London* 50 (1982): 1–28.
25. A. Dobson and J. Foufopoulos, "Emerging Infectious Pathogens of Wildlife," *Philosophical Transactions of the Royal Society of London, Series B*, 356 (2001): 1001–1012.
26. C. D. Harvell, K. Kim, J. M. Burkholder et al., "Emerging Marine Diseases: Climate Links and Anthropogenic Factors," *Science* 285 (1999): 1505–1510.
27. R. Stone, "Canine Virus Blamed in Caspian Seal Deaths," *Science* 289 (2000): 2017–2018.
28. M. A. Miller, I. A. Gardner, C. Kreuder et al., "Coastal Freshwater Runoff Is a Risk Factor for *Toxoplasma gondii* Infection of Southern Sea Otters (*Enhydra lutris nereis*)," *International Journal for Parasitology* 32 (2002): 997–1006.
29. N. D. Wolfe, A. A. Escalante, W. B. Karesh et al., "Wild Primate Populations in Emerging Infectious Disease Research: The Missing Link?" *Emerging Infectious Diseases* 4 (1998): 149–158; J. Wallis and D. R. Lee, "Primate Conservation: The Prevention of Disease Transmission," *International Journal of Primatology* 20 (1999): 803–826; D. Ferber, "Human Diseases Threaten Great Apes," *Science* 289 (2000): 1277–1278.
30. M. T. Oughton, H. L. N. Dick, B. M. Willey et al., "Methicillin-resistant *Staphylococcus aureus* as a Cause of Infections in Domestic Animals: Evidence for a New Humanotic Disease?" Presented at the American College for Microbiology, December 2001.
31. Dobson and Foufopoulos, "Emerging Infectious Pathogens of Wildlife."
32. L. H. Taylor, S. M. Latham, and M. E. J. Woolhouse, "Risk Factors for Human Disease Emergence," *Philosophical Transactions of the Royal Society of London, Series B*, 356 (2001): 983–989.
33. S. Cleaveland, M. K. Laurenson, and L. H. Taylor, "Diseases of Humans and Their Domestic Mammals: Pathogen Characteristics, Host Range, and the Risk of Emergence," *Philosophical Transactions of the Royal Society of London, Series B*, 356 (2001): 991–999.
34. Taylor et al., "Risk Factors."
35. F. A. Murphy, "Emerging Zoonoses," *Emerging Infectious Diseases* 4 (1998): 429–435.
36. Taylor et al., "Risk Factors."
37. Cleaveland et al., "Diseases of Humans."

38. ProMED-mail, "Avian Influenza, Human: East Asia," January 29, 2004.

39. Joshua Lederberg, Robert E. Shope, and Stanley C. Oaks, eds., *Emerging Infections: Microbial Threats to Health in the United States* (Washington, D.C.: National Academy Press, 1992), 43.

40. Cleaveland et al., "Diseases of Humans."

41. E. C. Holmes, "Molecular Epidemiology and Evolution of Emerging Infectious Diseases," *British Medical Bulletin* 54 (1998): 533–543.

42. R. M. Krause, quoted in Charles Greenblatt and Mark Spigelman, eds., *Emerging Pathogens* (New York: Oxford University Press, 2003), vii.

CHAPTER 2. Heirloom Infections:
Microbes before the Advent of Humans

1. Ronald Hare, *Pomp and Pestilence: Infectious Disease, Its Origins and Conquest* (London: Camelot Press, 1973), 33; Frank Ryan, *The Forgotten Plague* (Boston: Little, Brown, 1992), 4.

2. J. F. A. Sprent, "Evolutionary Aspects of Immunity in Zooparasitic Infections," in G. J. Jackson, ed., *Immunity to Parasitic Animals* (New York: Appleton, 1964), 3–64.

3. A. Cockburn, "Where Did Our Infectious Diseases Come From? The Evolution of Infectious Disease," in Ciba Foundation Symposium 49 (new series), *Health and Disease in Tribal Societies* (New York: Elsevier/Excerpta Medica/North-Holland, 1977), 103–113.

4. Richard Fiennes, *Zoonoses of Primates: The Epidemiology and Ecology of Simian Diseases in Relation to Man* (Ithaca: Cornell University Press, 1967), 67–68.

5. R. Hare, "The Antiquity of Diseases Caused by Bacteria and Viruses: A Review of the Problem from a Bacteriologist's Point of View," 128, in D. Brothwell and A. T. Sandison, eds., *Diseases in Antiquity* (Springfield, Ill.: Charles C. Thomas, 1967), 115–131.

6. D. J. McGeoch and A. J. Davison, "The Molecular Evolutionary History of the Herpesviruses," 459, in E. Domingo, R. Webster, and J. Holland, eds., *Origin and Evolution of Viruses* (New York: Academic Press, 1999), 441–465; see also D. J. McGeoch, S. Cook, A. Dolan et al., "Molecular Phylogeny and Evolutionary Timescale for the Family of Mammalian Herpesviruses," *Journal of Molecular Biology* 247 (1995): 443–458.

7. B. H. Robertson, "Viral Hepatitis and Primates: Historical and Molecular Analysis of Human and Nonhuman Primate Hepatitis A, B, and the GB-related Viruses," *Journal of Viral Hepatitis* 8 (2001): 233–242.

8. R. E. Lanford, D. Chavez, K. M. Brasky et al., "Isolation of a Hepadnavirus from the Woolly Monkey, a New World Primate," *Proceedings of the National Academy of Sciences USA* 95 (1998): 5757–5761; X. Hu, H. S. Margolis, R. H. Purcell et al., "Identification of Hepatitis B Virus Indigenous to Chimpanzees," *Proceedings of the National Academy of Sciences USA* 97 (2000): 1661–1664.

9. Richard Fiennes, *Zoonoses and the Origins and Ecology of Human Disease* (New York: Academic Press, 1978), 10–12.

10. D. J. Conway, C. Fanello, J. M. Lloyd et al., "Origin of *Plasmodium falciparum* Malaria Is Traced by Mitochondrial DNA," *Molecular and Biochemical Parasitology* 111 (2000): 163–171; McMichael, *Human Frontiers*, 79.

11. F.E.G. Cox, "Babesiosis and Malaria," in S. R. Palmer, E. J. L. Soulsby, and D.I.H. Simpson, eds., *Zoonoses: Biology, Clinical Practice, and Public Health Control* (New York: Oxford, 1998), 604.

12. Michael B. A. Oldstone, *Viruses, Plagues, and History* (New York: Oxford, 1998), 51.

13. W. W. Stead, "Genetics and Resistance to Tuberculosis: Could Resistance Be Enhanced by Genetic Engineering?" *Annals of Internal Medicine* 116 (1992):937–941.

CHAPTER 3. Humans as Hunters: Animal Origins of Bioterrorism

1. Jane van Lawick Goodall, *In the Shadow of Man* (Boston: Houghton Mifflin, 1971), 198–199, 281–282.
2. Donald Johnson and Maitland Edey, *Lucy: The Beginnings of Humankind* (New York: Simon and Schuster, 1981), 358.
3. McMichael, *Human Frontiers*, 47.
4. Ibid., 44, 47–48.
5. M. P. Richards, P. B. Pettitt, E. Trinkaus et al., "Neanderthal Diet at Vindija and Neanderthal Predation: The Evidence from Stable Isotopes," *Proceedings of the National Academy of Sciences* 97 (2000): 7663–7666.
6. S. B. Eaton and M. Konner, "Paleolithic Nutrition: A Consideration of Its Nature and Current Implications," *New England Journal of Medicine* 312 (1985): 283–289.
7. Eaton and Kenner, "Paleolithic Nutrition."
8. Richard Klein, *The Dawn of Human Culture* (New York: John Wiley and Sons, 2002).
9. Frans De Waal, *The Ape and the Sushi Master* (New York: Basic Books, 2001), 63.
10. J.-P. Rigaud, "Lascaux Cave: Art Treasures from the Ice Age," *National Geographic* 174 (1988): 482–499.
11. K. Turner, "Art with a Dark Past," *Washington Post*, July 30, 2000.
12. Miguel Angel Garcia Guinea, *Altamira and Other Cantabrian Caves* (Madrid: Silex, 2001), 46.
13. Garcia Guinea, *Altamira*, 64.
14. E. P. Hoberg, N. L. Alkire, A. de Queiroz et al., "Out of Africa: Origins of the *Taenia* Tapeworms in Humans," *Proceedings of the Royal Society of London, Series B* 268 (2001): 781–787.
15. H. H. Garcia, E. J. Pretell, R. H. Gilman et al., "A Trial of Antiparasitic Treatment to Reduce the Rate of Seizures due to Cerebral Cysticercosis," *New England Journal of Medicine* 350 (2004): 249–258.
16. A. C. Evans, M. B. Markus, R. J. Mason et al., "Late Stone-Age Coprolite Reveals Evidence of Prehistoric Parasitism" (letter), *South African Medical Journal* 86 (1996): 274–275.
17. "Human Anthrax Associated with an Epizootic among Livestock: North Dakota, 2000," *Morbidity and Mortality Weekly Report* 50 (2001): 677–680.
18. C. D. McGilvray, "The Transmission of Glanders from Horse to Man," *Journal of the American Veterinary Medical Association* 104 (1944): 255–263.
19. "The Civil War Quartermaster's Glanders Stable," http://www.lynchburgbiz.com/occ/Glanders/glanders.html, accessed December 10, 2003.
20. G. T. Sharrer, "The Great Glanders Epizootic, 1861–1866: A Civil War Legacy," *Agricultural History* 69 (1995): 79–97.
21. M. Quigley, "Veterinary Medicine and the American Civil War," *Veterinary Heritage* 24 (2001): 33–37.
22. Sharrer, "The Great Glanders Epizootic."
23. M. Rosenbloom, J. B. Leikin, S. N. Vogel et al., "Biological and Chemical Agents: A Brief Synopsis," *American Journal of Therapeutics* 9 (2002): 5–14.
24. Madeline Drexler, *Secret Agents: The Menace of Emerging Infections* (New York: Penguin Books, 2002), 236, 237.
25. T. J. Marrie, "Q Fever," in S. R. Palmer, E.J.L. Soulsby, and D.I.H. Simpson, eds., *Zoonoses: Biology. Clinical Practice and Public Health Control* (New York: Oxford, 1998), 180.
26. Jules Witcover, *Sabotage at Black Tom: Imperial Germany's Secret War in America, 1914–1917* (Chapel Hill: Algonquin Books, 1989), 126–127.
27. H. J. McGeorge II, "Chemical and Biological Terrorism: Analyzing the Problem," *ASA Newsletter* 42 (1994): 1, 12–13.

28. Witcover, *Sabotage at Black Tom*, 137.
29. Henry Landau, *The Enemy Within: The Inside Story of German Sabotage in America* (New York: G. P. Putnam's Sons, 1937); M. Wheelis, "First Shots Fired in Biological Warfare," *Nature* 395 (1998): 213.
30. Witcover, *Sabotage at Black Tom*, 248.
31. Landau, *The Enemy Within*, 194.
32. J. Bender, "Animals and Bioterrorism," http://www.cvm.umn.edu/anhlth_foodsafety/ Bioagroterrorism.pdf, accessed November 14, 2002.
33. C. Howe and W. R. Miller, "Human Glanders: Report of Six Cases," *Annals of Internal Medicine* 26 (1947): 93–115.
34. A. Srinivasan, C. N. Kraus, D. DeShazer et al., "Glanders in a Military Research Microbiologist," *New England Journal of Medicine* 345 (2001): 256–258; C. Georgiades and E. K. Fishman, "Glanders Disease of the Liver and Spleen: CT Evaluation," *Journal of Computer Assisted Tomography* 25 (2001): 91–93.

CHAPTER 4. Humans as Farmers: Microbes Move into the Home

1. A. Vekua, D. Lordkipanidze, G. P. Rightmire et al., "A new Skull of Early *Homo* from Dmanisi, Georgia," *Science* 297 (2002): 85–89.
2. McMichael, *Human Frontiers*, 188.
3. Ibid., 137.
4. Steve Olson, *Mapping Human History* (New York: Houghton Mifflin, 2003), 100.
5. S. Lev-Yadun, A. Gopher, and S. Abbo, "The Cradle of Agriculture," *Science* 288 (2000): 1602–1603.
6. Sonia Cole, *The Neolithic Revolution* (London: British Museum, 1970), 4–20.
7. Mark Nathan Cohen, *Health and the Rise of Civilization* (New Haven: Yale University Press, 1989), 22.
8. Cole, *The Neolithic Revolution*, 4, 38.
9. William H. McNeil, *Plagues and People* (New York: Anchor Books, 1977), 57.
10. Francis Galton, "The First Steps Towards the Domestication of Animals," *Transactions of the Ethnological Society of London*, N.S. 3, 122–138, quoted in *Juliet* Clutton-Brock, *Domesticated Animals from Early Times* (Austin: University of Texas Press, 1981), 15–16, 25.
11. P. Savolainen, Y. Zhang, J. Luo et al., "Genetic Evidence for an East Asian Origin of Domestic Dogs," *Science* 298 (2002): 1610–1613.
12. Stephen Budiansky, *The Covenant of the Wild: Why Animals Chose Domestication* (New York: William Morrow, 1992), 96.
13. Clutton-Brock, *Domesticated Animals*, 12.
14. Stephen Budiansky, *The Truth about Dogs* (New York: Penguin Books, 2000), 24.
15. Budiansky, *The Covenant of the Wild*, 24.
16. Rudyard Kipling, "The Cat That Walked by Himself," in *Just So Stories for Little Children* (New York: Weathervane Books, 1978), 170.
17. Cole, *The Neolithic Revolution*, 25; Clutton-Brock, *Domesticated Animals*, 56; M. A. Zeder and B. Hesse, "The Initial Domestication of Goats (*capra hircus*) in the Zagros Mountains 10,000 Years Ago," *Science* 287 (2000): 2254–2257.
18. Clutton-Brock, *Domesticated Animals*, 57–58.
19. E. Pennisi, "Horses Domesticated Multiple Times," *Science* 291 (2001): 412.
20. D. Perkins Jr., "Fauna of Çatal Hüyük: Evidence for Early Cattle Domestication in Anatolia," *Science* 164 (1969): 177–179.
21. Frederick E. Zeuner, *A History of Domesticated Animals* (London: Hutchinson, 1963), 240–241.
22. Clutton-Brock, *Domesticated Animals*, 84.
23. C. Vilà, J. A. Leonard, A. Götherström et al., "Widespread Origins of Domestic Horse Lineages," *Science* 291(2001): 474–477.

24. Jared Diamond, *The Third Chimpanzee* (New York: HarperCollins, 1992), 237.
25. Clutton-Brock, *Domesticated Animals*, 26.
26. Cole, *The Neolithic Revolution*, 21.
27. James Serpell, *In the Company of Animals* (Oxford: Basil Blackwell, 1986), 5.
28. Nancy K. Sandars, *Prehistoric Art in Europe* (London: Penguin Books, 1985), 435.
29. Keith Thomas, *Man and the Natural World: A History of Modern Sensibility* (New York: Pantheon Books, 1983), 95, 96.
30. Joanna Swabe, *Animals, Disease, and Human Society* (New York: Routledge, 1998), 51.
31. Paul G. Bahn, *The Cambridge Illustrated History of Prehistoric Art* (Cambridge: Cambridge University Press, 1998).
32. R. E. Pounder, "*Helicobacter pylori* and NSAIDs: The End of the Debate?" *Lancet* 358 (2002): 3–4.
33. M. Kidd and I. M. Modlin, "A Century of *Helicobacter pylori*," *Digestion* 59 (1998): 1–15.
34. S. Suerbaum and P. Michetti, "*Helicobacter pylori* Infection," *New England Journal of Medicine* 347 (2002): 1175–1186.
35. M. A. Mendall, P. M. Goggin, N. Molineaux et al., "Childhood Living Conditions and *Helicobacter pylori* Seropositivity in Adult Life," *Lancet* 339 (1992): 896–897.
36. S. Dimola and M. L. Caruso, "*Helicobacter pylori* in Animals Affecting the Human Habitat through the Food Chain," *Anticancer Research* 19 (1999): 3889–3894.
37. J. G. Fox, "Non-human Reservoirs of *Helicobacter pylori*," *Alimentary Pharmacology and Therapeutics* 9 (supp. 2) (1995): 93–103.
38. M. P. Dore, M. Bilotta, D. Vaira et al., "High Prevalence of *Helicobacter pylori* Infection in Shepherds," *Digestive Diseases and Sciences* 44 (1999): 1161–1164.
39. M. P. Dore, A. R. Sepulveda, H. El-Zimaity et al., "Isolation of *Helicobacter pylori* from Sheep: Implications for Transmission to Humans," *American Journal of Gastroenterology* 96 (2001): 1396–1401.
40. M. P. Dore, H. M. Malaty, D. Y. Graham et al., "Risk Factors Associated with *Helicobacter pylori* Infection among Children in a Defined Geographic Area," *Clinical Infectious Diseases* 35 (2002): 240–245.
41. M. P. Dore and D. Vaira, "Sheep Rearing and *Helicobacter pylori* Infection: An Epidemiological Model of Anthropozoonosis," *Digestive and Liver Disease* 35 (2003): 7–9; K. J. Goodman, P. Correa, H. J. Tenganá Aux et al., "*Helicobacter pylori* Infection in the Colombian Andes: A Population-Based Study of Transmission Pathways," *American Journal of Epidemiology* 144 (1996): 290–299.
42. Dore, Sepulveda et al., "Isolation of *Helicobacter pylori*."
43. A. van der Zee, H. Groenendijk, M. Peeters et al., "The Differentiation of *Bordetella parapertussis* and *Bordetella bronchiseptica* from Humans and Animals as Determined by DNA Polymorphism Mediated by Two Different Insertion Sequence Elements Suggests Their Phylogenetic Relationship," *International Journal of Systematic Bacteriology* 46 (1996): 640–647.
44. J. M. Musser, D. A. Bemis, H. Ishikawa et al., "Clonal Diversity and Host Distribution in *Bordetella bronchiseptica*," *Journal of Bacteriology* 169 (1987): 2793–2803; B. Arico, R. Gross, J. Smida et al., "Evolutionary Relationships in the Genus *Bordetella*," *Molecular Microbiology* 1 (1987): 301–308; M. Müller and A. Hildebrandt, "Nucleotide Sequences of the 23S rRNA Genes from *Bordetella pertussis, B. parapertussis, B. bronchiseptica*, and *B. avium*, and Their Implications for Phylogenetic Analysis," *Nucleic Acids Research* 21 (1993): 3320.
45. McNeil, *Plagues and People*, 257.
46. N. Douglass and K. Dumbell, "Independent Evolution of Monkeypox and Variola Viruses," *Journal of Virology* 66 (1992): 7565–7567; S. N. Shchelkunov, A. V. Totmenin, I. V. Babkin et al., "Human Monkeypox and Smallpox Viruses: Genomic Comparison," *FEBS Letters* 509 (2001): 66–70, 2001.

47. D. Baxby and M. Bennett, "Cowpox: A Re-evaluation of the Risks of Human Cowpox Based on New Epidemiological Information," *Archives of Virology* (supp.) 13 (1997): 1–12.

48. R. M. Kolhapure, R. P. Deolankar, C. D. Tupe et al., "Investigation of Buffalopox Outbreaks in Maharashtra State during 1992–1996," *Indian Journal of Medical Research* 106 (1997): 441–446.

49. Zeuner, *A History of Domesticated Animals*, 251.

50. R. Hare, "The Antiquity of Diseases Caused by Bacteria and Viruses: A Review of the Problem from a Bacteriologist's Point of View," 128, in D. Brothwell and A. T. Sandison, eds., *Diseases in Antiquity* (Springfield, Ill.: Charles C. Thomas, 1967), 127.

51. T. R. Frieden, T. R. Sterling, S. S. Munsiff et al., "Tuberculosis," *Lancet* 362 (2003): 887–899.

52. John Bunyan, *The Life and Death of Mr. Badman*, 1680, quoted in Rene Dubos and Jean Dubos, *The White Plague: Tuberculosis, Man and Society* (Boston: Little, Brown, 1952; New Brunswick, N.J.: Rutgers University Press, 1987, repr. 1996), 8.

53. A. Scorpio, D. Collins, D. Whipple et al., "Rapid Differentiation of Bovine and Human Tubercle Bacilli Based on a Characteristic Mutation in the Bovine Pyrazinamidase Gene," *Journal of Clinical Microbiology* 35 (1997): 106–110.

54. T. Garnier, K. Eiglmeier, J.-C. Camus et al., "The Complete Genome Sequence of *Mycobacterium bovis*," *Proceedings of the National Academy of Sciences USA* 100 (2003): 7877–7882.

55. M. Gutiérrez, S. Samper, M. Soledad Jiménez et al., "Identification by Spoligotyping of a Carpine Genotype in *Mycobacterium bovis* Strains Causing Human Tuberculosis," *Journal of Clinical Microbiology* 35 (1997): 3328–3330.

56. L. E. Espinosa de los Monteros, J. C. Galán, M. Gutiérrez et al., "Allele-Specific PCR Method Based on *pncA* and *oxyR* Sequences for Distinguishing *Mycobacterium bovis* from *Mycobacterium tuberculosis*: Intraspecific *M. bovis pncA* Sequence Polymorphism," *Journal of Clinical Microbiology* 36 (1998): 239–242.

57. Jacob Van der Hoeden, *Zoonoses* (Amsterdam, N.Y.: Elsevier, 1964), 22; J. H. Steele and A. F. Ranney, "Animal Tuberculosis," *American Review of Tuberculosis and Pulmonary Diseases* 77 (1958): 908–922.

58. Van der Hoeden, *Zoonoses*, 15.

59. Aidan Cockburn, *The Evolution and Eradication of Infectious Diseases* (Baltimore: Johns Hopkins University Press, 1963), 221.

60. Steele and Ranney, "Animal Tuberculosis."

61. L. F. Ayvazian, "History of Tuberculosis," in L. B. Reichman and E. S. Hershfield, eds., *Tuberculosis: A Comprehensive International Approach* (New York: Marcel Dekker, 1993), 2.

62. Mirko D. Grmek, *Diseases of the Ancient Greek World* (Baltimore: Johns Hopkins University Press, 1989), 193. W. L. Salo, A. C. Aufderheide, J. Buikstra et al., "Identification of *Mycobacterium tuberculosis* DNA in a Pre-Columbian Peruvian Mummy," *Proceedings of the National Academy of Sciences USA* 91 (1994): 2091–2094.

63. Thomas M. Daniel, *Captain of Death: The Story of Tuberculosis* (Rochester, N.Y.: University of Rochester Press, 1997), 24.

64. Frederick F. Cartwright and Michael Biddiss, *Disease and History*, 2nd ed. (Stroud, England: Sutton, 2000), 137.

65. Lee B. Reichman and Janice H. Tanne, *Timebomb: The Global Epidemic of Multi-Drug-Resistant Tuberculosis* (New York: McGraw Hill, 2002), 17.

66. Daniel, *Captain of Death*, 25.

67. Reichman and Tanne, *Timebomb*, 16.

68. Daniel, *Captain of Death*, 30.

69. Dubos and Dubos, *The White Plague*, 9.

70. René Dubos, *Mirage of Health: Utopias, Progress, and Biological Change* (New York: Harper, 1959), 204.

71. Daniel, *Captain of Death*, 104, quoting W. Hale-White, *Keats as Doctor and Patient* (London: Oxford, 1938), no page given; 105, quoting W. A. Wells, *A Doctor's Life of John Keats* (New York: Vantage Press, 1959), 1198–1199.
72. John Keats, *Ode to a Nightingale*, 1820, www.bbc.co.uk/nature/poetry/nightingale .shtml, accessed December 15, 2003.
73. Daniel, *Captain of Death*, 34.
74. Edgar Allan Poe, "The Masque of the Red Death," 1842, http://bau2.uibk.ac.at/sg/poe/works/reddeath.html, accessed December 15, 2003.
75. Dubos and Dubos, *The White Plague*, 19.
76. Lewis J. Moorman, *Tuberculosis and Genius* (Chicago: University of Chicago Press, 1940), 21, 17.
77. D. H. Lawrence, "The Ship of Death," 1928, in R. Aldington, ed., *Last Poems* (London: Martin Secker, 1933), http://eir.library.utoronto.ca/rpo/display/poem1251.html, accessed December 15, 2003.
78. Frieden et al., "Tuberculosis."
79. S. E. Kline, L. L. Hedemark, and S. F. Davies, "Outbreak of Tuberculosis among Regular Patrons of a Neighborhood Bar," *New England Journal of Medicine* 333 (1995): 222–227.
80. C. R. Braden and the Investigative Team, "Infectiousness of a University Student with Laryngeal and Cavitary Tuberculosis." *Clinical Infectious Diseases* 21 (1995): 565–570.
81. "Public Health Dispatch: Tuberculosis Outbreak among Homeless Persons—King County, Washington, 2002–2003," *Morbidity and Mortality Weekly Report* 52 (2003): 1209–1210.

Chapter 5. Humans as Villagers: Microbes in the Promised Land

1. Karlen, *Man and Microbes*, 25.
2. Cole, *The Neolithic Revolution*, 55–56 (see chap. 4, n. 6).
3. F. Fenner, "Sociocultural Change and Environmental Diseases," in N. F. Stanley and R. A. Joske, eds., *Changing Disease Patterns and Human Behaviour* (New York: Academic Press, 1980).
4. Glyn Daniel, *The First Civilizations* (New York: Thomas Y. Crowell, 1968), 69.
5. Colin McEvedy, *The Penguin Atlas of Ancient History* (Baltimore: Penguin Books, 1967), 26.
6. Karlen, *Man and Microbes*, 52.
7. Cohen, *Health*, 117 (see chap. 4, n. 7).
8. McMichael, *Human Frontiers*, 377 (see chap. 1, n. 8).
9. M. J. Rodrigo and J. Dopazo, "Evolutionary Analysis of the Picornavirus Family," *Journal of Molecular Evolution* 40 (1995): 362–371.
10. Andrew Cliff, Peter Haggett, and Matthew Smallman-Raynor, *Measles: An Historical Geography of a Major Human Viral Disease* (Oxford: Blackwell, 1993), 46.
11. Cliff et al., *Measles*, xiii, 4.
12. Oldstone, *Viruses, Plagues, and History*, 76–77 (see chap. 2, n. 12).
13. F. A. Gibbs, E. L. Gibbs, P. R. Carpenter et al., "Electroencephalographic Abnormality in 'Uncomplicated' Childhood Diseases," *Journal of the American Medical Association* 171 (1959): 1050–1055.
14. Oldstone, *Viruses, Plagues, and History*, 78–79.
15. T. Barrett and P. B. Rossiter, "Rinderpest: The Disease and Its Impact on Humans and Animals," *Advances in Virus Research* 53 (1999): 89–110; M. Shiotani, R. Miura, K. Fujita et al., "Molecular Properties of the Matrixprotein (M) Gene of the Lapinized Rinderpest Virus," *Journal of Veterinary Medical Science* 63 (2001): 801–805; K. M. Westover and A. L. Hughes, "Molecular Evolution of Viral Fusion and Ma-

trix Protein Genes and Phylogenetic Relationships among the Paramyxoviridae," *Molecular Phylogenetics and Evolution* 21 (2001): 128–134; T. Barrett, I.K.G. Visser, L. Mamaev et al., "Dolphin and Porpoise Morbilliviruses Are Genetically Distinct from Phocine Distemper Virus," *Virology* 193 (1993): 1010–1012.

16. Thomas, *Man and the Natural World,* 94, 95.
17. On Al-Razi and Fuller, Cliff et al., *Measles,* 52, 61.
18. Karlen, *Man and Microbes,* 102.
19. McNeil, *Plagues and People,* 219.
20. P. J. Bianchine and T. A. Russo, "The Role of Epidemic Infectious Diseases in the Discovery of America," *Allergy Proceedings* 13 (1992): 225–232.
21. Karlen, *Man and Microbes,* 103.
22. McNeil, *Plagues and People,* 212–213.
23. Cliff et al., *Measles,* 65.
24. McNeil, *Plagues and People,* 213–214.
25. Cliff et al., *Measles,* 113.
26. R. J. Wolfe, "Alaska's Great Sickness,1900: An Epidemic of Measles and Influenza in a Virgin Soil Population," *Proceedings of the American Philosophical Society* 126 (1982): 91–121.
27. Cliff et al., *Measles,* 116–117.
28. Ibid., 85, 211–212.
29. Ibid., 125–126, 127.
30. Oldstone, *Viruses, Plagues, and History,* 74.
31. Cliff et al., *Measles,* 133.
32. Ibid., 104.
33. Oldstone, *Viruses, Plagues, and History,* 81, 80, found in Robert E. Lee, *The War of the Rebellion: A Compilation of the Official Records of the Union and Confederate Armies.* (Washington, D.C., 1880–1902), 657.
34. Cliff et al., *Measles,* 103, 104.
35. Margaret Mitchell, *Gone with the Wind* (New York: Macmillan, 1936), 134–135.

CHAPTER 6. Humans as Traders: Microbes Get Passports

1. Daniel, *The First Civilizations,* 72.
2. McMichael, *Human Frontiers,* 178; C. S. Troy, D. E. MacHugh, J. F. Bailey et al., "Genetic Evidence for Near-Eastern Origins of European Cattle," *Nature* 410 (2001): 1088–1091.
3. Martin, "Earth History" (see chap. 1, n. 14).
4. McMichael, *Human Frontiers,* 103.
5. 2 Sam. 24:15
6. Is. 37:36.
7. Archeology, Online News, Nikos Axarlis, "Plague Victims Found: Mass Burial in Athens," http://www.archaeology.org/online/news/kerameikos.html, accessed April 15, 1998.
8. R. S. Bray, *Armies of Pestilence: The Impact of Disease on History* (New York: Barnes and Noble Books), 7.
9. L. L. Jacobs and D. Pilbeam, "Of Mice and Men: Fossil-Based Divergence Dates and Molecular 'Clocks,'" *Journal of Human Evolution* 9 (1980): 551–555.
10. Zinsser, *Rats, Lice, and History,* 192 (see chap. 1, n. 15).
11. M. Achtman, K. Zurth, G. Morelli et al., "*Yersinia pestis,* the Cause of Plague, Is a Recently Emerged Clone of *Yersinia pseudotuberculosis,*" *Proceedings of the National Academy of Sciences USA* 96 (1999): 14043–14048.
12. M. B. Prentice, K. D. James, J. Parkhill et al., "*Yersinia pestis* pFra Shows Biovar-Specific Differences and Recent Common Ancestry with a *Salmonella enterica* Serovar Typhi Plasmid," *Journal of Bacteriology* 183 (2001): 2586–2594.

13. Edward Marriott, *Plague: A Story of Science, Rivalry, and a Scourge That Won't Go Away* (New York: Henry Holt, 2002), 252.
14. C. LeDuff, "Up, Down, In, and Out in Beverly Hills," *New York Times*, September 17, 2002.
15. Karlen, *Man and Microbes*, 75.
16. Bray, *Armies of Pestilence*, 23.
17. Zinsser, *Rats, Lice and History*, 199.
18. William Shakespeare, *Hamlet* 3.4.23, in William G. Clark and William A. Wright, eds., *The Complete Works of William Shakespeare* (London: Spring Books, n.d.), 966.
19. Miguel de Cervantes, *Don Quixote de la Mancha*, 4.10. 319.
20. Barbara Tuchman, *A Distant Mirror: The Calamitous Fourteenth Century* (New York: Alfred A. Knopf, 1978), 93.
21. Norman F. Cantor, *In the Wake of the Plague: The Black Death and the World It Made* (New York: Free Press, 2001), 172.
22. Tuchman, *A Distant Mirror*, 92.
23. John Findlay Drew Shrewsbury, *A History of Bubonic Plague in the British Isles* (Cambridge: Cambridge University Press, 1971), 21.
24. Giovanni Boccaccio, *The Decameron*, M. Rigg, trans., vol. 1 (London: David Campbell, 1921), 5–11. (http://www.fordham.edu/halsall/source/boccacio2.html).
25. Petrarch quoted in Cartwright and Biddiss, *Disease and History*, 40.
26. Tuchman, *A Distant Mirror*, 94.
27. Cantor, *In the Wake of the Plague*, 157.
28. Tuchman, *A Distant Mirror*, 94.
29. Ibid., 95.
30. Shrewsbury, *A History*, 93.
31. *Annals of Ireland*, quoted in Shrewsbury, *A History*, 47.
32. Cantor, *In the Wake of the Plague*, 6.
33. Shrewsbury, *A History*, 480.
34. Dubos, *Mirage of Health*, 157 (see chap. 4, n. 70).
35. An excellent account of the San Francisco epidemic can be found in Marilyn Chase, *The Barbary Plague: The Black Death in Victorian San Francisco* (New York: Random House, 2003).
36. "Pneumonic Plague: Arizona, 1992," *Morbidity and Mortality Weekly Report* 41 (1992): 739.
37. C. M. Vega and T. Kelley, "Couple from New Mexico Remain Hospitalized in New York with Plague," *New York Times*, November 9, 2002.
38. LeDuff, "Up, Down, In and Out."
39. ProMED-mail, "Plague: Algeria (Oran) (04)," July 4, 2003.
40. LeDuff, "Up, Down, In and Out."
41. J. Gillis, "A Nose for Gene Data," *Washington Post*, January 21, 2002.
42. Marriott, *Plague*, 231.
43. J.-C. Affray, E. Tchernov, and E. Nevo, "Origine du commensalisme de la souris domestique (Mus musculus domesticus) vis-à-vis de l'homme," *Comptes Rendus Acad Sci* 307 (1988): 517–522.
44. N. Nathanson and S. Nichol, "Korean Hemorrhagic Fever and Hantavirus Pulmonary Syndrome: Two Examples of Emerging Hantaviral Diseases," in R. Krause, ed., *Emerging Infections: Biomedical Research Reports* (New York: Academic Press, 2000), 371.
45. ProMED-mail, "Hantavirus Pulmonary Syndrome: USA (New Mexico)," December 5, 2003.
46. J. N. Mills, A. Corneli, J. C. Young et al., "Hantavirus Pulmonary Syndrome: United

States: Updated Recommendations for Risk Reduction," *Morbidity and Mortality Weekly Report* 51 [RR-9] (2002): 1–5.
47. Nathanson and Nichol, "Korean Hemorrhagic Fever," 369.

CHAPTER 7. Humans as Pet Keepers: Microbes Move into the Bedroom

The chapter epigraph is from Martin, "Earth History."
 1. Zeuner, *A History of Domesticated Animals*, 108 (see chap. 4, n. 21).
 2. J. A. Serpell, "The Domestication and History of the Cat," in D. C. Turner and P. Bateson, eds., *The Domestic Cat* (Cambridge: Cambridge University Press, 1988), 154.
 3. Serpell, *In the Company of Animals*, 34–37 (see chap. 4, n. 27).
 4. Swabe, *Animals, Disease and Human Society*, 162–163 (see chap. 4, n. 30).
 5. Thomas, *Man and the Natural World*, 103–104 (see chap. 4, no. 29).
 6. Ibid.
 7. William Shakespeare, *Cymbeline*, 2.1.7; *The Merchant of Venice*, 4.1.133; *The Tempest*, 1.1.21, in William G. Clark and William A. Wright, eds., *The Complete Works of William Shakespeare* (London: Spring Books, n.d.).
 8. Thomas, *Man and the Natural World*, 105.
 9. Swabe, *Animals, Disease, and Human Society*, 158.
 10. "The Middle Ages," http://62.108.6.218/~roos/dotkom/pages/frames_eng/dogs_history.html, © 1996 Melody Underwood Hobbs, revised February 1997, accessed August 29, 2002.
 11. Budiansky, *The Truth about Dogs*, 34 (see chap. 4, n. 14).
 12. Kathleen Kete, *The Beast in the Boudoir: Petkeeping in Nineteenth-Century Paris* (Berkeley: University of California Press, 1994), 53, 33.
 13. Zeuner, *A History of Domesticated Animals*, 396.
 14. Kete, *The Beast in the Boudoir*, 124.
 15. Harriet Ritvo, *The Animal Estate* (Cambridge: Harvard University Press, 1987), 129.
 16. Kete, *The Beast in the Boudoir*, 115.
 17. Frances Simpson, *The Book of the Cat* (New York: Cassell, 1903), 14.
 18. William Rush, "Thoughts on Insanity," *Knick* 7 (1836): 33–36.
 19. J. L. Lynnlee, *Purrrfection: The Cat* (West Chester, Pa.: Schiffer, 1990), 26–28.
 20. Lyn Murfin, *Popular Leisure in the Lake Counties* (Manchester: Manchester University Press, 1990), 14. Kete, *The Beast in the Boudoir*, 3.
 21. A. Repplier, "Agrippina," *Atlantic Monthly* 69 (1892): 753–763.
 22. A. M. Beck and N. M. Myers, "Health Enhancement and Companion Animal Ownership," *Annual Review of Public Health* 17 (1996): 247–257.
 23. Swabe, *Animals, Disease, and Human Society*, 187.
 24. Forbes.com, Markets: PETsMART, Inc., http://www.forbes.com/finance/mktguideapps/compinfo/CompanyTearsheet.jhtml?repno=A07E3, accessed March 17, 2003; Yahoo! Finance, "Petco Quarterly Earnings Rise 36 Percent," http://biz.yahoo.com/rb/030313/retail_petco_earns_2.html, accessed March 17, 2003.
 25. B. R. Hundley, "Introduction to Market Size," from abstract of a paper presented at the South African Society for Animal Science Conference, July 2000, www.afma.co.za/AFMA_Template/1,2491,6552_1645,00.html, accessed October 28, 2002.
 26. J. Pomfret, "Dog Fight Bares Marks of Civil Society in China," *Washington Post*, December 3, 2000. A. A. Avery, "U.S. Farming in the 21st Century," *Proceedings, Southern Weed Science Society 2002*, lxxvii.
 27. "Fun Pet Statistics," American Pet Association, www.apapets.com/petstats2.htm, accessed October 28, 2002; E. F. Torrey and R. H. Yolken, "A Survey of Infectious Agents in Cats and Their Owners," unpublished, 2003; F. Kunkle, "A Swanky Spa Where Fur Is De Rigueur," *Washington Post*, December 22, 2002.

28. Kunkle, "A Swanky Spa."
29. C. Loose, "Travels with Cinnamon," *Washington Post*, October 12, 2003; J. Miller, "Take Your Pet on Vacation," *Washington Post*, June 8, 2003.
30. Kunkle, "A Swanky Spa."
31. B. Bilger, "The Last Meow," *New Yorker*, September 8, 2003, 46–53.
32. M. Mott, "Cat Cloning Offered to Pet Owners," http://news.nationalgeographic.com/ news/2004/03/0324_040324_catclones.html, accessed April 1, 2004.
33. "In the Company of Dogs" catalog, Spring 2003 (P.O. Box 3330, Chelmsford, MA 01824-0955), 2, 36; "Care-A-Lot Pet Supply Warehouse" catalog, Holiday 2002 (1617 Diamond Springs Rd., Virginia Beach, VA 23455), 3, 64.
34. "Critters," *Seattle Times*, December 25, 2002.
35. "Pet Memorials," www.ferretstore.com/pet-memorials.html, accessed June 16, 2003.
36. Bilger, "The Last Meow"; "Gross National Product by Country: 1990 and 2000," in *Statistical Abstract of the United States: 2002* (Washington, D.C.: U.S. Government Printing Office, 2002), 833.
37. M. Rich, "Pet Therapy Sets Landlords Howling," *New York Times*, June 26, 2003.
38. M. Sink, "Colorado: Pets as Companions," *New York Times*, February 11, 2003.
39. K. Allen and J. Blascovich, "The Value of Service Dogs for People with Severe Ambulatory Disabilities," *Journal of the American Medical Association* 275 (1996): 1001–1006.
40. J. M. Siegel, F. J. Angulo, R. Detels et al., "AIDS Diagnosis and Depression in the Multicenter AIDS Cohort Study: The Ameliorating Impact of Pet Ownership," *AIDS Care* 11 (1999): 157–170.
41. Rich, "Pet Therapy."
42. L. K. Bustad and L. M. Hines, "Placement of Animals with the Elderly: Benefits and Strategies," in A. H. Katcher and A. M. Beck, eds., *New Perspectives on Our Lives with Companion Animals* (Philadelphia: University of Pennsylvania Press, 1983), 291.
43. M. M. Baun and B. W. McCabe, "Companion Animals and Persons with Dementia of the Alzheimer's Type," *American Behavioral Scientist* 47 (2003): 42–51.
44. K. M. Allen, J. Blascovich, J. Tomaka et al., "Presence of Human Friends and Pet Dogs as Moderators of Autonomic Responses to Stress in Women," *Journal of Personality and Social Psychology* 61 (1991): 582–589.
45. R. L. Zasloff and A. H. Kidd, "Loneliness and Pet Ownership among Single Women," *Psychological Reports* 75 (1994): 747–752.
46. A. H. Kidd and R. M. Kidd, "Benefits and Liabilities of Pets for the Homeless," *Psychological Reports* 74 (1994): 715–722. B. Williams, "Dogs in Words: Quotes about Canines," American Kennel Club Web site, http://wwwakc.org/life/words/quotes.cfm, accessed July 7, 2003.
47. Allen et al., "Presence of Human Friends"; K. Allen, J. Blascovich, and W. B. Mendes, "Cardiovascular Reactivity and the Presence of Pets, Friends, and Spouses: The Truth about Cats and Dogs," *Psychosomatic Medicine* 64 (2002): 727–739.
48. E. Friedmann, A. H. Katcher, J. J. Lynch et al., "Animal Companions and One-Year Survival of Patients after Discharge from a Coronary Care Unit," *Public Health Reports* 95 (1980): 307–312; E. Friedmann and S. A. Thomas, "Pet Ownership, Social Support, and One-Year Survival after Acute Myocardial Infarction in the Cardiac Arrhythmia Suppression Trial (CAST)," *American Journal of Cardiology* 76 (1995): 1213–1217.
49. J. Serpell, "Beneficial Effects of Pet Ownership on Some Aspects of Human Health and Behaviour," *Journal of the Royal Society of Medicine* 84 (1991): 717–720.
50. J. M. Siegel, "Stressful Life Events and Use of Physician Services among the Elderly: The Moderating Role of Pet Ownership," *Journal of Personality and Social Psychology* 58 (1990): 1081–1086.
51. B. M. Levinson, "The Dog as a 'Co-Therapist,'" *Mental Hygiene* 46 (1962): 59–65.

52. J. Riedler, C. Braun-Fahrländer, W. Eder et al., "Exposure to Farming in Early Life and Development of Asthma and Allergy: A Cross-Sectional Survey," *Lancet* 358 (2001): 1129–1133.

53. D. R. Ownby, C. Cole Johnson, and E. L. Peterson, "Exposure to Dogs and Cats in the First Year of Life and Risk of Allergic Sensitization at 6 to 7 Years of Age," *Journal of the American Medical Association* 288 (2002): 963–972.

54. McNeil, *Plagues and People*, 70 (see chap. 4, n. 9).

55. D. A. Talan, D. M. Citron, F. M. Abrahamian et al., for the Emergency Medicine Animal Bite Infection Study Group, "Bacteriologic Analysis of Infected Dog and Cat Bites," *New England Journal of Medicine* 340 (1999): 85–92.

56. Talan et al., "Bacteriologic Analysis."

57. E.J.C. Goldstein, "Household Pets and Human Infections," *Infectious Disease Clinics of North America* 5 (1991): 117–130.

58. M. Plaut, E. M. Zimmerman, and R. A. Goldstein, "Health Hazards to Humans Associated with Domestic Pets," *Annual Review of Public Health* 17 (1996): 221–245.

59. D. G. McNeil Jr., "Hundreds of U.S. Troops Infected by Parasite Borne by Sand Flies, Army Says," *New York Times*, December 6, 2003.

60. R. S. Desowitz, *Who Gave Pinta to the Santa Maria?* (New York: W. W. Norton, 1997), 40.

61. R. Fisa, M. Gállego, S. Castillejo et al., "Epidemiology of Canine Leishmaniasis in Catalonia (Spain): The Example of the Priorat Focus," *Veterinary Parasitology* 83 (1999): 87–97; J. Moreno and J. Alvar, "Canine Leishmaniasis: Epidemiological Risk and the Experimental Model," *Trends in Parasitology* 18 (2002): 399–405.

62. D. W. Chen, "A New Epidemic Proves Fatal to 21 Foxhounds," *New York Times*, August 25, 2000, http://www.remnantofgod.org/nat-142.htm, accessed September 4, 2002.

63. R. B. Tesh, "Ecological Sources of Zoonotic Diseases," in T. Burroughs, S. Knobler, and J. Lederberg, eds., *The Emergence of Zoonotic Diseases* (Washington, D.C.: National Academy Press, 2002), 44–45.

64. ProMED-mail, "Leptospirosis, Fatal—USA: Background," April 12, 2004, accessed at http://www.promedmail.org.

65. ProMED-mail, "Rabies, Human: China (Nationwide)," November 25, 2003.

66. P. M. Schantz, "Of Worms, Dogs, and Human Hosts: Continuing Challenges for Veterinarians in Prevention of Human Disease," *Journal of the American Veterinary Medical Association* 204 (1994): 1023–1028.

67. I. D. Robertson and R. C. Thompson, "Enteric Parasitic Zoonoses of Domesticated Dogs and Cats," *Microbes and Infection* 4 (2002): 867–873.

68. A. Steiner, "Environmental Studies on Multiple Sclerosis," *Neurology* 2 (1952): 260–262. S. D. Cook and P. C. Dowling, "A Possible Association between House Pets and Multiple Sclerosis," *Lancet* 1 (1977): 980–982.

69. S. Jotkowitz, "Multiple Sclerosis and Exposure to House Pets" (letter), *Journal of the American Medical Association* 238 (1977): 854. M. Alter, M. Berman, and E. Kahana, "The Year of the Dog," *Neurology* 29 (1979): 1023–1026.

70. S. D. Cook, C. Rohowsky-Kochan, S. Bansil et al., "Evidence for Multiple Sclerosis as an Infectious Disease," *Acta Neurologica Scandinavica Suppl* 161 (1995): 34–42.

71. Cook et al., "Evidence for Multiple Sclerosis."

72. S. D. Cook and P. C. Dowling, "Distemper and Multiple Sclerosis in Sitka, Alaska," *Annals of Neurology* 11 (1982): 192–194.

73. M. J. Hodge and C. Wolfson, "Canine Distemper Virus and Multiple Sclerosis," *Neurology* 49 (supp. 2) (1997): S62–S69.

74. J. D. Kravetz and D. G. Federman, "Cat-Associated Zoonoses," *Archives of Internal Medicine* 162 (2002): 1945–1952.

75. K. L. Gage, D. T. Dennis, K. A. Orloski et al., "Cases of Cat-Associated Human Plague

in the Western US, 1977–1998," *Clinical Infectious Diseases* 30 (2000): 893–900. See also M. Eidson, L. A. Tierney, O. J. Rollag et al., "Feline Plague in New Mexico: Risk Factors and Transmission to Humans," *American Journal of Public Health* 78 (1988): 1333–1335.

76. S. Uga, T. Minami, and K. Nagata, "Defecation Habits of Cats and Dogs and Contamination by *Toxocara* Eggs in Public Park Sandpits," *American Journal of Tropical Medicine and Hygiene* 54 (1996): 122–126.

77. G. Desmonts, J. Couvreur, F. Alison et al., "Etude Épidémiologique sur la Toxoplasmose: De l'Influence de la Cuisson des Viands de Boucherie sur la Fréquence de l'Infection Humaine," *Revue Française d'Études Cliniques et Biologiques* 10 (1965): 952–958.

78. G. D. Wallace, "Experimental Transmission of *Toxoplasma gondii* by Filth-Flies," *American Journal of Tropical Medicine and Hygiene* 20 (1971): 411–413. G. D. Wallace, "Experimental Transmission of *Toxoplasma gondii* by Cockroaches," *Journal of Infectious Diseases* 126 (1972): 545–547.

79. J. P. Dubey and C. P. Beattie, *Toxoplasmosis of Animals and Man* (Boca Raton, Fla.: CRC Press, 1988), 120.

80. G. Kapperud, P. A. Jenum, B. Stray-Pedersen et al., "Risk Factors for *Toxoplasma gondii* Infection in Pregnancy: Results of a Prospective Case-Control Study in Norway," *American Journal of Epidemiology* 144 (1996): 405–412.

81. J. L. Jones, D. Kruszon-Moran, M. Wilson et al., "*Toxoplasma gondii* Infection in the United States: Seroprevalence and Risk Factors," *American Journal of Epidemiology* 154 (2001): 357–365.

82. G. Desmonts and J. Couvreur, "Toxoplasmosis in Pregnancy and Its Transmission to the Fetus," *Bulletin of the New York Academy of Medicine* 50 (1974): 144–159.

83. J. K. Frenkel and A. Ruiz, "Human Toxoplasmosis and Cat Contact in Costa Rica," *American Journal of Tropical Medicine and Hygiene* 29 (1980): 1167–1180.

84. C. Soto, "Toxoplasmosis in Pregnancy," *Clinician Reviews* 12 (2002): 51–56.

85. W. Kramer, "Frontiers of Neurological Diagnosis in Acquired Toxoplasmosis," *Psychiatria, Neurologia, Neurochirurgia* 69 (1966): 43–64.

86. D. M. Israelski and J. S. Remington, "Toxoplasmic Encephalitis in Patients with AIDS," *Infectious Disease Clinics of North America* 2 (1988): 429–445.

87. G. N. Holland, "Reconsidering the Pathogenesis of Ocular Toxoplasmosis," *American Journal of Ophthalmology* 128 (1999): 502–505; Israelski and Remington, "Toxoplasmic Encephalitis."

88. Israelski and Remington, "Toxoplasmic Encephalitis."

89. P.-A. Witting, "Learning Capacity and Memory of Normal and *Toxoplasma*-Infected Laboratory Rats and Mice," *Zeitschrift für Parasitenkunde* 61 (1979): 29–51; G. Piekarski, "Behavioral Alterations Caused by Parasitic Infection in Case of Latent Toxoplasma Infection," *Zentralblatt für Bakteriologie, Mikrobiologie und Hygiene. 1. Abt. Originale A* 250 (1981): 403–406.

90. J. P. Webster, "Rats, Cats, People, and Parasites: The Impact of Latent Toxoplasmosis on Behaviour," *Microbes and Infection* 3 (2001): 1037–1045.

91. E. M. Betin, "Concerning the Study of Toxoplasmosis in Mentally Disturbed Patients," *Zhurnal nevropatologii i psikhiatrii imeni S.S. Korsakova* 69 (1969): 909–913; P. Bossi, E. Caumes, L. Paris et al., "*Toxoplasma gondii*–Associated Guillain-Barré Syndrome in an Immunocompetent Patient," *Journal of Clinical Microbiology* 36 (1998): 3724–3725; P. Ryan, S. F. Hurley, A. M. Johnson et al., "Tumours of the Brain and Presence of Antibodies to *Toxoplasma gondii*," *International Journal of Epidemiology* 22 (1993): 412–419.

92. J. Flegr and J. Havlíček, "Changes in the Personality Profile of Young Women with Latent Toxoplasmosis," *Folia Parasitologica* 46 (1999): 22–28; J. Havlíček, Z. Gašová, A. P. Smith et al., "Decrease of Psychomotor Performance in Subjects with Latent

'Asymptomatic' Toxoplasmosis," *Parasitology* 122 (2001): 515–520; J. Flegr, M. Preiss, J. Klose et al., "Decreased Level of Psychobiological Factor Novelty Seeking and Lower Intelligence in Men Latently Infected with the Protozoan Parasite *Toxoplasma gondii:* Dopamine, a Missing Link between Schizophrenia and Toxoplasmosis?" *Biological Psychiatry* 63 (2003): 253–268.

93. Kramer, "Frontiers of Neurological Diagnosis." See also E. Aeffner, L. Schmidtke, H. J. Seeberger et al., Kasuistischer Beitrag zur akuten Erwachsenen Toxoplasmose (Encephalitis, Myositis Ossificans, Symptomatische Psychose), *Nervenarzt* 26 (1955): 161–166; W. Kretschmer Jr. and E. E. Schmid, "Komplizierte Psychose bei Toxoplasma-Encephalitis," *Archiv für Psychiatrie und Nervenkrankheiten* 193 (1955): 38–47; A. Minto and F. J. Roberts, "The Psychiatric Complications of Toxoplasmosis," *Lancet* 1 (1959): 1180–1182.

94. E. F. Torrey and R. H. Yolken, "*Toxoplasma gondii* and Schizophrenia," *Emerging Infectious Diseases* 9 (2003): 1375–1380.

95. S. L. Buka, R. H. Yolken, E. F. Torrey et al., "Viruses, Fetal Hypoxia, and Subsequent Schizophrenia: A Direct Test of Infectious Agents Using Prenatal Sera (Abstract)," *Schizophrenia Research* 36 (1999): 38.

96. E. F. Torrey and R. H. Yolken, "Could Schizophrenia Be a Viral Zoonosis Transmitted from House Cats?" *Schizophrenia Bulletin* 21 (1995): 167–171; E. F. Torrey, R. Rawlings, and R. H. Yolken, "The Antecedents of Psychoses: A Case-Control Study of Selected Risk Factors," *Schizophrenia Research* 46 (2000): 17–23.

97. N. L. Gottlieb, N. Ditchek, J. Poiley et al., "Pets and Rheumatoid Arthritis: An Epidemiologic Survey," *Arthritis and Rheumatism* 17 (1974): 229–234.

98. C. Bond and L. G. Cleland, "Rheumatoid Arthritis: Are Pets Implicated in Its Etiology?" *Seminars in Arthritis and Rheumatism* 25 (1996): 308–317.

99. G. Morrison, "Zoonotic Infections from Pets: Understanding the Risks and Treatment," *Postgraduate Medicine* 110 (2001): 24–48.

100. Ibid.

101. K. Ryan-Poirier, P. Y. Whitehead, and R. J. Leggiadro, "An Unlucky Rabbit's Foot?" *Pediatrics* 85 (1990): 598–600; R. Horwick, "Tularemia Revisited," *New England Journal of Medicine* 345 (2001): 1637–1639.

102. D. Vanrompay, R. Ducatelle, and F. Haesebrouck, "*Chlamydia psittaci* Infections: A Review with Emphasis on Avian Chlamydiosis," *Veterinary Microbiology* 45 (1995): 93–119.

103. B. Crosse, "Psittacosis: A Clinical Review," *Journal of Infection* 21 (1990): 251–259.

104. J. F. Moroney, R. Guevara, C. Iverson et al., "Detection of Chlamydiosis in a Shipment of Pet Birds, Leading to Recognition of an Outbreak of Clinically Mild Psittacosis in Humans," *Clinical Infectious Diseases* 26 (1998): 1425–1429.

105. Moroney et al., "Detection of Chlamydiosis."

106. I. Ito, T. Ishida, M. Mishima et al., "Familial Cases of Psittacosis: Possible Person-to-Person Transmission," *Internal Medicine* 41 (2002): 580–583.

107. D. W. Gregory and W. Schaffner, "Psittacosis," *Seminars in Respiratory Infections* 12 (1997): 7–11.

108. P. E. Verweij, J.F.G.M. Meis, R. Eijk et al., "Severe Human Psittacosis Requiring Artificial Ventilation: Case Report and Review," *Clinical Infectious Diseases* 20 (1995): 440–442.

109. J. T. Kirchner, "Psittacosis," *Postgraduate Medicine* 102 (1997): 181–194.

110. Vanrompay et al., "*Chlamydia psittaci* Infections."

111. F. Bonnet, P. Morlat, I. Delevaux et al., "A Possible Association between *Chlamydiae psittacci* Infection and Temporal Arteritis," *Joint Bone Spine* 67 (2000): 550–552; Paul W. Ewald, *Plague Time: How Stealth Infections Can Cause Cancer, Heart Disease, and Other Deadly Ailments* (New York: Free Press, 2000), 123.

112. R. Ackerman, "Epidemiologic Aspects of Lymphocytic Choriomeningitis in Man," in

F. Lehmann-Grube, ed., *Lymphocytic Choriomeningitis Virus and Other Arenaviruses* (New York: Springer-Verlag, 1973), 233–237.

113. R. J. Biggar, J. P. Woodall, P. D. Walter et al., "Lymphocytic Choriomeningitis Outbreak Associated with Pet Hamsters: Fifty-seven Cases from New York State," *Journal of the American Medical Association* 232 (1975): 494–500.

114. M. S. Hirsch, R. C. Moellering Jr., H. G. Pope et al., "Lymphocytic-Choriomeningitis-Virus Infection Traced to a Pet Hamster," *New England Journal of Medicine* 291 (1974): 610–612.

115. J. Hotchin, E. Sikora, W. Kinch et al., "Lymphocytic Choriomeningitis in a Hamster Colony Causes Infection of Hospital Personnel," *Science* 185 (1974): 1173–1174. R. J. Biggar, T. J. Schmidt, and J. P. Woodall, "Lymphocytic Choriomeningitis in Laboratory Personnel Exposed to Hamsters Inadvertently Infected with LCM Virus," *Journal of the American Veterinary Medical Association* 171 (1977): 829–832.

116. G. M. Komrower, B. L. Williams, and P. B. Stones, "Lymphocytic Choriomeningitis in the Newborn: Probable Transplacental Infection," *Lancet* 1 (1955): 697–698; Biggar et al., "Lymphocytic choriomeningitis."

117. H. H. Skinner, E. H. Knight, and M. C. Lancaster, "Lymphomas Associated with a Tolerant Lymphocytic Choriomeningitis Virus Infection in Mice," *Laboratory Animals* 14 (1980): 117–121; M. Kohler, B. Rüttner, S. Cooper et al., "Enhanced Tumor Susceptibility of Immunocompetent Mice Infected with Lymphocytic Choriomeningitis Virus," *Cancer Immunology, Immunotherapy* 32 (1990): 117–124.

118. J. Ginsburg, "Dinner, Pets, and Plagues by the Bucketful," http://www.the-scientist.com/yr2004/apr/research2_040412.html, accessed June 2, 2004.

119. S. Hartwell, "The American Feral Cat Problem," 1994, accessed November 5, 2002, at http://messybeast.com/usferal.htm.

120. J. Gorman, "Bird Lovers Hope to Keep Cats on a Very Short Leash," *New York Times*, March 18, 2003.

121. Dobson and Foufopoulos, "Emerging Infectious Pathogens" (see chap. 1, n. 25).

122. "Petting Zoo Directory," www.pettingzoofarm.com, accessed November 26, 2002.

123. Zoo-to-You Web site, www.zoo-to-you.com/page5.htm, accessed November 26, 2002.

124. "In College Football, a Struggle for Fans," *New York Times*, November 23, 2002.

125. J. A. Crump, A. C. Sulka, A. J. Langer et al., "An Outbreak of *Escherichia coli* O157:H7 Infections among Visitors to a Dairy Farm," *New England Journal of Medicine* 347 (2002): 555–560.

126. "Outbreaks of *Escherichia coli* O157:H7 Infections among Children Associated with Farm Visits: Pennsylvania and Washington, 2000," *Morbidity and Mortality Weekly Report* 50 (2001): 293–297.

127. "*Inside Edition* Investigates Petting Zoos to Report on Possible Dangers for Some Children When They Are Exposed to Bacteria from Farm Animals," aired May 6, 2002, www.insideedition.com/investigative/pet-zoo.htm, accessed November 26, 2002.

128. A. L. Cowan, "Drawing a Line at Pets with Long Scaly Tails," *New York Times*, April 25, 2003.

129. D. Oldenburg, "Born to Be Wild," *Washington Post*, July 30, 2003.

130. "National Alternative Pet Association," http://www.altpet.net, accessed June 16, 2003.

131. C. E. Rupprecht, J. Gilbert, K. R. Marshall et al., "Evaluation of an Inactivated Rabies Virus Vaccine in Domestic Ferrets," *Journal of the American Veterinary Medical Association* 196 (1990): 1514–1616.

132. C. L. Besch-Williford, "Biology and Medicine of the Ferret," *Veterinary Clinics of North America: Small Animal Practice* 17 (1987): 1155–1183; R. P. Marini, J. A. Adkins, and J. G. Fox, "Proven or Potential Zoonotic Diseases of Ferrets," *Journal of the American Veterinary Medical Association* 195 (1989): 990–994.

133. "NYPD Officer: Tranquilized Tiger Came at Me," *CNN.com/U.S.*, October 6, 2003, http://www.cnn.com/2003/US/Northeast/10/06/cnna.duffy/index.html.

134. "Price List and Availability," Exotic Pets 4 Sale Web site, http://members.tripod.com/ladysreddragon/id24_m.htm, accessed June 16, 2003.

135. "Family Keeps Pet Eel in Tub for 33 Years," *USA Today*, January 8, 2003, 4A.

136. B. B. Chomel, "Less Common House Pets," in D. Schlossberg, ed., *Infections of Leisure* (Washington, D.C.: American Society for Microbiology, 1999), 238.

137. "Reptile-Associated Salmonellosis: Selected States, 1998–2002," *Morbidity and Mortality Weekly Report* 52 (2003): 1206–1209.

138. A. Goodnough, "Forget the Gators: Exotic Pets Run Wild in Florida," *New York Times*, February 29, 2004.

139. Cowan, "Drawing a Line."

140. "Reptile-Associated Salmonellosis: Selected States, 1994–1995," *Morbidity and Mortality Weekly Report* 44 (1995): 347–350.

141. D. M. Ackman, P. Drabkin, G. Birkhead et al., "Reptile-Associated Salmonellosis in New York State," *Pediatric Infectious Disease Journal* 14 (1995): 955–959.

142. "Reptile-Associated Salmonellosis: Selected States, 1996–1998."

143. D. L. Woodward, R. Khakhria, and W. M. Johnson, "Human Salmonellosis Associated with Exotic Pets," *Journal of Clinical Microbiology* 35 (1997): 2786–2790.

144. "Reptile-associated Salmonellosis—Selected States, 1996–1998," *Morbidity and Mortality Weekly Report* 48 (1999): 1009–1013.

145. Woodward et al., "Human salmonellosis associated with exotic pets."

146. "Iguana-Associated Salmonellosis: Indiana, 1990," *Morbidity and Mortality Weekly Report* 41 (1992): 38–39.

147. C. Dalton, R. Hoffman, and J. Pape, "Iguana-Associated Salmonellosis in Children," *Pediatric Infectious Disease Journal* 14 (1995): 319–320.

148. J. Mermin, B. Hoar, and F. J. Angulo, "Iguanas and *Salmonella marina* Infection in Children: A Reflection of the Increasing Incidence of Reptile-Associated Salmonellosis in the United States," *Pediatrics* 99 (1997): 399–402.

149. G. J. Moran, "Dogs, Cats, Raccoons, and Bats: Where Is the Real Risk for Rabies?" *Annals of Emergency Medicine* 39 (2002): 541–543.

150. A. Dobson, "Raccoon Rabies in Space and Time," *Proceedings of the National Academy of Sciences* 97 (2000): 14041–14043.

151. S. R. Jenkins, B. D. Perry, and W. G. Winkler, "Ecology and Epidemiology of Raccoon Rabies," *Reviews of Infectious Diseases* 10 (supp. 4) (1988): S620–S625; V. F. Nettles, "Rabies in Translocated Raccoons," *American Journal of Public Health* 69 (1979): 601–602.

152. Jenkins et al., "Ecology and Epidemiology."

153. "Rabies in a Beaver: Florida, 2001," *Morbidity and Mortality Weekly Report* 51 (2002): 481–482.

154. B. A. Woodruff, J. L. Jones, and T. R. Eng, "Human Exposure to Rabies from Pet Wild Raccoons in South Carolina and West Virginia, 1987 through 1988," *American Journal of Public Health* 81 (1991): 1328–1330.

155. L. D. Rotz, J. A. Hensley, C. E. Rupprecht et al., "Large-Scale Human Exposures to Rabid or Presumed Rabid Animals in the United States: 22 Cases (1990–1996)," *Journal of the American Veterinary Medical Association* 212 (1998): 1198–1200.

156. "First Human Death Associated with Raccoon Rabies: Virginia, 2003," *Morbidity and Mortality Weekly Report* 52 (2003): 1102–1103.

157. J. Wilgoren, "Monkeypox Casts Light on Rule Gap for Exotic Pets," *New York Times*, June 10, 2003.

158. ProMED-mail, "International Animal Movement: Veterinary Control," June 11, 2003.

159. "The African Gambian Pouch Rat," Petite Paws Exotics, http://members.shaw.ca/petitepaws/gpr.html, accessed June 16, 2003.
160. ProMED-mail, "Monkeypox, Human, Prairie Dogs: USA (12)," June 19, 2003. See also K. D. Reed, J. W. Melski, M. B. Graham et al., "The Detection of Monkeypox in Humans in the Western Hemisphere," *New England Journal of Medicine* 350 (2004): 342–350.

CHAPTER 8. Humans as Diners: Mad Cows and Sane Chickens

1. Drexler, *Secret Agents*, 113 (see chap. 3, n. 24).
2. "Hepatitis A Outbreak Associated with Green Onions at a Restaurant: Monaca, Pennsylvania," *Morbidity and Mortality Weekly Report*, 52 (2003): 1–3.
3. "Preliminary FoodNet Data on the Incidence of Foodborne Illnesses: Selected Sites, United States, 2002," *Morbidity and Mortality Weekly Report*, 52 (2003): 340–343.
4. V. J. Cirillo, "Fever and Reform: The Typhoid Epidemic in the Spanish-American War," *Journal of the History of Medicine* 55 (2000): 363–397.
5. P. S. Mead, L. Slutsker, V. Dietz et al., "Food-Related Illness and Death in the United States," *Emerging Infectious Diseases* 5 (1999): 607–625.
6. U.S. Department of Agriculture, *Salmonella Enteritidis Risk Assessment: Shell Eggs and Egg Products* (Washington, D.C.: USDA Food Safety and Inspection Service, 1998), http://www.fsis.usda.gov/ophs/risk, accessed August 13, 2002; J. M. Cowden, "Salmonellosis and Eggs: Public Health, Food Poisoning, and Food Hygiene," *Current Opinion in Infectious Diseases* 3 (1990): 246–249; D. C. Rodrigue, R. V. Tauxe, and B. Rowe, "International Increase in *Salmonella enteritidis*: A New Pandemic?" *Epidemiology and Infection* 105 (1990): 21–27.
7. W. C. Levine, J. F. Smart, D. L. Archer et al., "Foodborne Disease Outbreaks in Nursing Homes," *Journal of the American Medical Association* 266 (1991): 2105–2109; B. Mishu, J. Koehler, L. A. Lee et al., "Outbreaks of *Salmonella enteritidis* Infections in the United States, 1985–1991," *Journal of Infectious Diseases* 169 (1994): 547–552.
8. S. Umasankar, E. U. Mridha, M. M. Hannan et al., "An Outbreak of *Samonella enteritidis* in a Maternity and Neonatal Intensive Care Unit," *Journal of Hospital Infection* 34 (1996): 117–122.
9. U.S. Department of Agriculture, *Salmonella Enteritidis Risk Assessment.*
10. "Outbreak of Multidrug-Resistant *Salmonella Newport*: United States, January–April 2002," *Journal of the American Medical Association* 288 (2002): 951–953.
11. M. Helms, P. Vastrup, P. Gerner-Smidt et al., "Excess Mortality Associated with Antimicrobial Drug-Resistant *Salmonella typhimurium*," *Emerging Infectious Diseases* 8 (2002): 490–495.
12. S. M. Graham, "Salmonellosis in Children in Developing and Developed Countries and Populations," *Current Opinion in Infectious Diseases* 15 (2002): 507–512.
13. U.S. Department of Agriculture, Food Safety and Inspection Service, "Proposed Rules," *Federal Register* 63 (96) (1998): 27502–27511, http://www.fsis.usda.gov/OPPDE/rdad/FRPubs/96-035A.pdf, accessed August 13, 2002.
14. "Outbreaks of *Salmonella* Serotype *enteritidis* Infection Associated with Eating Shell Eggs: United States, 1999–2001," *Morbidity and Mortality Weekly Report* 51 (2003): 1149–1152.
15. E. F. Coyle, S. R. Palmer, C. D. Ribeiro et al., "*Salmonella enteritidis* Phage Type 4 Infection: Associated with Hens' Eggs," *Lancet* 2 (1988): 1295–1297.
16. Cowden, "Salmonellosis and Eggs."
17. Coyle et al., "*Salmonella enteritidis.*"
18. B. Mishu, P. M. Griffin, R. V. Tauxe et al., "*Salmonella enteritidis* Gastroenteritis Transmitted by Intact Chicken Eggs," *Annals of Internal Medicine* 115 (1991): 190–194.

19. Cowden, "Salmonellosis and Eggs."
20. S. L. Mawer, G. E. Spain, and B. Rowe, "*Salmonella enteritidis* Phage Type 4 and Hens' Eggs" (letter), *Lancet* 1 (1989): 280–281.
21. U.S. Department of Agriculture, Food Safety and Inspection Service, "Proposed Rules."
22. E. A. Ager, K. E. Nelson, M. M. Galton et al., "Two Outbreaks of Egg-Borne Salmonellosis and Implications for Their Prevention," *Journal of the American Medical Association* 199 (1967): 372–378.
23. Ibid.
24. Cowden, "Salmonellosis and Eggs."
25. C. W. Hedberg, M. J. David, K. E. White et al., "Role of Egg Consumption in Sporadic *Salmonella enteritidis* and *Salmonella typhimurium* Infections in Minnesota," *Journal of Infectious Diseases* 167 (1993): 107–111.
26. M. E. St. Louis, D. L. Morse, M. E. Potter et al., "The Emergence of Grade A Eggs as a Major Source of *Salmonella enteritidis* Infections," *Journal of the American Medical Association* 259 (1988): 2103–2107.
27. A. S. Kessel, I. A. Gillespie, S. J. O'Brien et al., "General Outbreaks of Infectious Intestinal Disease Linked with Poultry, England and Wales, 1992–1999," *Communicable Disease and Public Health* 4 (2001): 171–177.
28. T. Kistemann, F. Dangendorf, L. Krizek et al., "GIS-Supported Investigation of a Nosocomial *Salmonella* Outbreak," *International Journal of Hygiene and Environmental Health* 203 (2000): 117–126.
29. S. Sivapalasingam, E. Barrett, A. Kimura et al., "A Multistate Outbreak of *Salmonella enterica* Serotype *Newport* Infection Linked to Mango Consumption: Impact of Water-Dip Disinfestations Technology," *Clinical Infectious Diseases* 37 (2003): 1585–1590.
30. "Salmonellosis Associated with Chicks and Ducklings: Michigan and Missouri, Spring 1999," *Morbidity and Mortality Weekly Report* 49 (2000): 297–299.
31. "*Salmonella hadar* Associated with Pet Ducklings: Connecticut, Maryland, and Pennsylvania, 1991," *Morbidity and Mortality Weekly Report* 41 (1992): 185–187, in *Journal of the American Medical Association* 267 (1992): 2011.
32. H. J. Shivaprasad, "Fowl Typhoid and Pullorum Disease," *Revue Scientifique et Technique (International Office of Epizootics)* 19 (2000): 405–424.
33. J. Li, N. H. Smith, K. Nelson et al., "Evolutionary Origin and Radiation of the Avian-Adapted Non-motile Salmonellae," *Journal of Medical Microbiology* 38 (1993): 129–139.
34. W. Rabsch, B. M. Hargis, R. M. Tsolis et al., "Competitive Exclusion of *Salmonella enteritidis* by *Salmonella gallinarum* in Poultry," *Emerging Infectious Diseases* 6 (2000): 443–448; A. J. Bäumler, B. M. Hargis, and R. M. Tsolis, "Tracing the Origins of *Salmonella* Outbreaks," *Science* 287 (2000): 50–52.
35. Rodrigue et al., "International Increase."
36. U.S. Department of Agriculture, Food Safety and Inspection Service, "Proposed Rules."
37. U.S. Department of Agriculture, *Salmonella Enteritidis Risk Assessment.*
38. P. A. Barrow, "The Paratyphoid Salmonellae," *Revue Scientifique et Technique (International Office of Epizootics)* 19 (2000): 351–375.
39. Kessel et al., "General Outbreaks."
40. C. S. DeWaal, "Playing Chicken: The Human Cost of Inadequate Regulation of the Poultry Industry," Food Safety Program, Center for Science in the Public Interest, March 1996, http://www.cspinet.org/reports/polt.html, accessed July 30, 2002.
41. "Chicken: What You Don't Know Can Hurt You," *Consumer Reports*, March 1998, 7.
42. Kessel et al., "General Outbreaks."
43. S. I. Miller, E. L. Hohmann, and D. A. Pegues, "*Salmonella* (Including *Salmonella typhi*)," in G. L. Mandell, J. E. Bennett, and R. Dolin, eds., *Principles and Practice of*

Infectious Diseases, 4th ed., vol. 2 (New York: Churchill Livingstone, 1995), 2013–2033.

44. "*Salmonella typhimurium* Outbreak in Sweden from Contaminated Jars of Helva (or Halva)," *Communicable Diseases Intelligence* 25 (2001): 183.

45. "Outbreak of Multidrug-Resistant *Salmonella Newport*: United States, January–April 2002," *Journal of the American Medical Association* 288 (2002): 951–953; ProMED-mail, "*Salmonella kiambu*, beef jerky: USA (New Mexico)," October 2, 2003.

46. P. C. Craven, D. C. Mackel, W. B. Baine et al., "International Outbreak of *Salmonella eastbourne* Infection Traced to Contaminated Chocolate," *Lancet* 1 (1975): 788–792.

47. D. N. Taylor, I. K. Wachsmuth, Y. Shangkuan et al., "Salmonellosis Associated with Marijuana: A Multistate Outbreak Traced by Plasmid Fingerprinting," *New England Journal of Medicine* 306 (1982): 1249–1253.

48. Mead et al., "Food-Related Illness."

49. W. H. van der Poel, J. Vinje, R. van der Heide et al., "Norwalk-like Calicivirus Genes in Farm Animals," *Emerging Infectious Diseases* 6 (2000): 36–41.

50. J. McLauchlin and N. Van der Mee-Marquet, "Listeriosis," in S. R. Palmer, E.J.L. Soulsby, and D.I.H. Simpson, eds., *Zoonoses: Biology, Clinical Practice, and Public Health Control* (Oxford: Oxford University Press, 1998), 127–140.

51. "Outbreak of Listeriosis: Northeastern United States, 2002," *Journal of the American Medical Association* 288 (2002): 2260.

52. E. Becker, "Consumer Groups Accuse U.S. of Negligence on Food Safety, Leading to Meat Recalls," *New York Times*, October 15, 2002.

53. M. B. Skirrow, "Campylobacteriosis," in S. R. Palmer, E.J.L. Soulsby, and D.I.H. Simpson, eds., *Zoonoses: Biology, Clinical Practice, and Public Health Control* (Oxford: Oxford University Press, 1998), 37–46.

54. M. Lecuit, E. Abachin, A. Martin et al., "Immunoproliferative Small Intestinal Disease Associated with *Campylobacter jejuni*," *New England Journal of Medicine* 350 (2004): 239–248.

55. Skirrow, "Campylobacteriosis."

56. G. M. Pupo, R. Lan, and P. R. Reeves, "Multiple Independent Origins of Shigella Clones of *Escherichia coli* and Convergent Evolution of Many of Their Characteristics," *Proceedings of the National Academy of Sciences USA* 97 (2000): 10567–10572.

57. S. Nelson, R. C. Clarke, and M. A. Karmali, "Verocytotoxin-Producing *Escherichia coli* (VTEC) Infections," in S. R. Palmer, E.J.L. Soulsby, and D.I.H. Simpson, eds., *Zoonoses: Biology, Clinical Practice, and Public Health Control* (Oxford: Oxford University Press, 1998), 89–104.

58. Ibid.

59. J. R. Brandt, L. S. Fouser, S. L. Watkins et al., "*Escherichia coli* O157:H7-Associated Hemolytic-Uremic Syndrome after Ingestion of Contaminated Hamburgers," *Journal of Pediatrics* 125 (1994): 519–526; B. P. Bell, M. Goldoft, P. M. Griffin et al., "A Multistate Outbreak of *Escherichia coli* O157:H7-Associated Bloody Diarrhea and Hemolytic Uremic Syndrome from Hamburgers: The Washington Experience," *Journal of the American Medical Association* 272 (1994): 1349–1353.

60. P. R. Cieslak, S. J. Noble, D. J. Maxson et al., "Hamburger-Associated *Escherichia coli* O157:H7 Infection in Las Vegas: A Hidden Epidemic," *American Journal of Public Health* 87 (1997): 176–180.

61. ProMED-mail, "*E. coli* 0157, Salad: USA (California)," October 10, 2003.

62. "Excerpts from the Agriculture Secretary's News Conference," *New York Times*, December 24, 2003.

63. ProMED-mail, "CJD (New Var.), Carrier Frequency Study—UK," May 21, 2004.

64. D. Grady, "Mad Cow Quandary: Making Animal Feed," *New York Times*, February 6, 2004.
65. N. Nathanson, K. A. McGann, J. Wilesmith et al., "The Evolution of Virus Diseases: Their Emergence, Epidemicity, and Control," *Virus Research* 29 (1993): 3–20.
66. S. Blakeslee and M. Burros, "Danger to Public Is Low, Experts on Disease Say," *New York Times*, December 24, 2003.
67. P. J. Bosque, "Bovine Spongiform Encephalopathy, Chronic Wasting Disease, Scrapie, and the Threat to Humans from Prion Disease Epizootics," *Current Neurology and Neuroscience Reports* 2 (2002): 488–495.
68. Z. Davanipour, M. Alter, E. Sobel et al., "Transmissible Virus Dementia: Evaluation of a Zoonotic Hypothesis," *Neuroepidemiology* 5 (1986): 194–206; E. D. Belay, P. Gambetti, L. B. Schonberger et al., "Creutzfeldt-Jakob Disease in Unusually Young Patients Who Consumed Venison," *Archives of Neurology* 58 (2001): 1673–1678.
69. N. Bons, N. Mestre-Frances, P. Belli et al., "Natural and Experimental Oral Infection of Nonhuman Primates by Bovine Spongiform Encephalopathy Agents," *Proceedings of the National Academy of Sciences USA* 96 (1999): 4046–4051.
70. ProMED-mail, "Feline Spongiform Encephalopathy, Cat: Switzerland," August 24, 2003.
71. G. Zanusso, E. Nardelli, A. Rosati et al., "Simultaneous Occurrence of Spongiform Encephalopathy in a Man and His Cat in Italy," *Lancet* 352 (1998): 1116–1118.
72. Blakeslee, "Mad Cows, Sane Cats" (see chap. 1, n. 1).
73. Henig, *A Dancing Matrix*, 111 (see chap. 1, n. 11).
74. "Study Examines Venison Eaters' Risk of Contracting Brain Disease," *Rocky Mountain News of Colorado*, July 1, 2002.
75. J. C. Bartz, R. F. Marsh, D. I. McKenzie et al., "The Host Range of Chronic Wasting Disease Is Altered on Passage in Ferrets," *Virology* 251 (1998): 297–301.

CHAPTER 9. Microbes from the Modern Food Chain: Lessons from SARS, Influenza, and Bird Flu

The epigraph quote is from Peter Cordingly, speaking for the World Health Organization on CNN, January 14, 2004.
1. R. G. Webster, "Wet Markets: A Continuing Source of Severe Acute Respiratory Syndrome and Influenza?" *Lancet* 363 (2004): 234–236.
2. ProMED-mail, "SARS Worldwide (164): Etiology," July 23, 2003.
3. F. Zeng, K.Y.C. Chow, and F. C. Leung, "Estimated Timing of the Last Common Ancestor of the SARS Coronavirus" (letter), *New England Journal of Medicine* 349 (2003): 2469–2470.
4. ProMED-mail, "SARS Worldwide (03): Etiology," January 6, 2004.
5. S.K.C. Ng, "Possible Role of an Animal Vector in the SARS Outbreak at Amoy Gardens," *Lancet* 362 (2003): 570–572.
6. Y. Ding, L. He, Q. Zhang et al., "Organ Distribution of Severe Acute Respiratory Syndrome (SARS) Associated Coronavirus (SARS-CoV) in SARS Patients: Implications for Pathogenesis and Virus Transmission Pathways," *Journal of Pathology* 203 (2004): 622–630.
7. J.S.M. Peiris, K. Y. Yuen, A.D.M.E. Osterhaus et al., "The Severe Acute Respiratory Syndrome," *New England Journal of Medicine* 349 (2003): 2431–2441.
8. P.C.Y. Woo, S.K.P. Lau, H. Tsoi et al., "Relative Rates of Non-pneumonic SARS Coronavirus Infection and SARS Coronavirus Pneumonia," *Lancet* 363 (2004): 841–845.
9. N. Wade, "New SARS Study Stresses Need to Act Fast against Epidemics," *New York Times*, January 30, 2004.

10. R. G. Webster, W. J. Bean, O. T. Gorman et al., "Evolution and Ecology of Influenza A Viruses," *Microbiological Reviews* 56 (1992): 152–179.
11. Y. Suzuki and M. Nei, "Origin and Evolution of Influenza Virus Hemagglutinin Genes," *Molecular Biology and Evolution* 19 (2002): 501–509.
12. Edwin D. Kilbourne, *Influenza* (New York: Plenum, 1987), 242.
13. C. Scholtissek and E. Naylor, "Fish Farming and Influenza Pandemics," *Nature* 331 (1988): 215.
14. McMichael, *Human Frontiers*, 147 (see chap. 1, n. 8).
15. I. H. Brown, "The Epidemiology and Evolution of Influenza Viruses in Pigs," *Veterinary Microbiology* 74 (2000): 29–46.
16. Webster et al., "Evolution and Ecology."
17. Lynette Iezzoni, *Influenza 1918* (New York: TV Books, 1999), 41.
18. William Ian Beveridge, *Influenza: The Last Great Plague*, rev. ed. (New York: Prodist, 1978), 25, 27.
19. Lederberg et al., *Emerging Infections*, 18 (see chap. 1, n. 39).
20. Alfred W. Crosby, *America's Forgotten Pandemic: The Influenza of 1918* (Cambridge: Cambridge University Press, 1990), 31.
21. A. H. Reid, T. G. Fanning, J. V. Hultin et al., "Origin and Evolution of the 1918 'Spanish' Influenza Virus Hemagglutinin Gene," *Proceedings of the National Academy of Sciences USA* 96 (1999): 1651–1656.
22. Crosby, *America's Forgotten Pandemic*, 53.
23. N. R. Grist, "Pandemic Influenza 1918" (letter written September 29, 1918), reprinted in *British Medical Journal* 2: 1632–1633, 1979, www.hibernianhealth.com/flu_letter .html, accessed July 3, 2002.
24. Crosby, *America's Forgotten Pandemic*, 140.
25. Ibid., 77, 82.
26. Iezzoni, *Influenza 1918*, 158.
27. Gina Kolata, *Flu: The Story of the Great Influenza Pandemic of 1918 and the Search for the Virus That Caused It* (New York: Touchstone, 1999), 53.
28. Crosby, *America's Forgotten Pandemic*, 324.
29. Ibid., 102, 105.
30. Iezzoni, *Influenza 1918*, 69.
31. Crosby, *America's Forgotten Pandemic*, 228.
32. Iezzoni, *Influenza 1918*, 167.
33. Mary McCarthy, *Memories of a Catholic Girlhood* (New York: Harcourt, Brace and World, 1946), 35.
34. Thomas Wolfe, *Look Homeward Angel* (New York: Collier Books, 1929), 488.
35. Crosby, *America's Forgotten Pandemic*, 317.
36. Katherine Anne Porter, *Pale Horse, Pale Rider* (New York: New American Library, 1936), 126.
37. J. Pickrell, "Killer Flu with a Human-Pig Pedigree?" *Science* 292 (2001): 1041.
38. R. G. Webster, "Influenza Virus: Transmission between Species and Relevance to Emergence of the Next Human Pandemic," *Archives of Virology* 13 (supp.) (1997): 105–113.
39. ProMED-mail, "Avian Influenza, WHO Fact Sheet," January 16, 2004.
40. ProMED-mail, "Avian Influenza, Human: East Asia (15)," February 6, 2004.
41. ProMED-mail, "Avian Influenza, Human: Vietnam (11)," January 22, 2004.
42. ProMED-mail, "Avian Influenza, Eastern Asia (72): Thailand," May 15, 2004.
43. M. S. Klempner and D. S. Shapiro, "Crossing the Species Barrier: One Small Step to Man, One Giant Leap to Mankind," *New England Journal of Medicine* 350 (2004): 1171–1172.
44. L. K. Altman, "Human Spread, a First, Is Suspected in Bird Flu in Vietnam," *New York Times*, February 2, 2004.

45. R. J. Webby and R. G. Webster, "Are We Ready for Pandemic Influenza?" *Science* 302 (2003): 1519–1522.
46. Editorial, "Avian Influenza: The Threat Looms," *Lancet* 363 (2004): 257.
47. ProMED-mail, "Avian Influenza H5N2, Poultry: USA (Texas)," February 21, 2004; Avian Influenza — Canada (23)," May 7, 2004.
48. Pérez-Peña and L. K. Altman, "With Rare Case of Avian Flu, a Troubling Medical Mystery," *New York Times*, April 20, 2004.
49. Webster, "Wet Markets."
50. ProMED-mail, "Avian Influenza: Eastern Asia (14)," January 30, 2004.

CHAPTER 10. The Coming Plagues: Lessons from AIDS, West Nile Virus, and Lyme Disease

1. Henig, *A Dancing Matrix*, xii (see chap. 1, n. 11).
2. ProMED-mail, accessed May to June 2003, at http://www.promedmail.org, archive numbers 20030522.1250 and 20030501.1088 (Venereal Disease), 20030630.1611 (Akabane Virus), 20030606.1391 and 20030503.1106 (Kyasanur Forest Disease), 20030527.1299 (Catarrhal Fever), 20030522.1254 (Trout Disease), 20030510.1161 (Gastroenteritis), 20030513.1190 (Bluetongue Virus Disease), 20030603.1350 (African Swine Fever), and 20030528.1305 (Avian Influenza).
3. E. Bailes, F. Gao, F. Bibollet-Ruche et al., "Hybrid Origin of SIV in Chimpanzees," *Science* 300 (2003): 1713.
4. J. I. Brooks, E. W. Rud, R. G. Pilon et al., "Cross-Species Retroviral Transmission from Macaques to Human Beings," *Lancet* 360 (2002): 387–388.
5. S. Van Dooren, M. Salemi, and A.-M. Vandamme, "Dating the Origin of the African Human T-Cell Lymphotropic Virus Type-1 (HTLV-1) Subtypes," *Molecular Biology and Evolution* 18 (2001): 661–671.
6. Diamond, *The Third Chimpanzee*, 23 (see chap. 4, n. 24).
7. D. M. Hillis, "Origins of HIV," *Science* 288 (2000): 1757–1760; B. Korber, M. Muldoon, J. Theiler et al., "Timing the Ancestor of the HIV-1 Pandemic Strains," *Science* 288 (2000): 1789–1796; N. D. Wolfe, W. M. Switzer, J. K. Carr et al., "Naturally Acquired Simian Retrovirus Infection in Central African Hunters," *Lancet* 363 (2004): 932–937.
8. Peter Lamptey, Merywen Wigley, Dara Carr, and Yvette Collymore, "*Facing the HIV/AIDS Pandemic*," *Population Bulletin*, vol. 57, no. 3 (Washington, D.C.: Population Reference Bureau, 2002), 1.
9. "Update: AIDS: United States, 2000," *Morbidity and Mortality Weekly Report* 51 (2002): 592–595. H. Jaffe, "Whatever Happened to the U.S. AIDS Epidemic?" *Science* 305 (2004): 1243–1244.
10. M. C. Layton, "Challenges of Vectorborne Disease Surveillance from the Local Perspective: West Nile Virus Experience," in T. Burroughs, S. Knobler, and J. Lederberg, eds., *The Emergence of Zoonotic Diseases: Understanding the Impact of Animal and Human Health* (Washington, D.C.: National Academy Press, 2002), 86–90.
11. M. Enserink, "New York's Lethal Virus Came from Middle East, DNA Suggests," *Science* 286 (1999): 1450–1451.
12. Dobson and Foufopoulos, "Emerging Infectious Pathogens of Wildlife" (see chap. 1, n. 25).
13. "Provisional Surveillance Summary of the West Nile Virus Epidemic: United States, January–November 2002," *Morbidity and Mortality Weekly Report* 51 (2002): 1129–1133.
14. D. Brown, "West Nile Virus Kills Four, Sickens 88 in Three States," *Washington Post*, August 3, 2002.

15. S. J. Olsen, H.-L. Chang, T. Yung-Yan Cheung et al., "Transmission of the Severe Acute Respiratory Syndrome on Aircraft," *New England Journal of Medicine* 349 (2003): 2416–2422.

16. International Civil Aviation Organization, ICAO Circular 291-AT/123, *The World of Civil Aviation, 2001–2004* (Montreal: ICAO, 2002), 27.

17. P. J. Irwin, "Companion Animal Parasitology: A Clinical Perspective," *International Journal of Parasitology* 32 (2002): 581–593.

18. ProMED-mail, "Exotic Disease Risk, Traveling pets—UK," May 18, 2004; "Exotic Disease Risk, Traveling Pets—UK (02)," May 19, 2004.

19. L. Simonsen, A. Kane, J. Lloyd et al., "Unsafe Injections in the Developing World and Transmission of Bloodborne Pathogens: A Review," *Bulletin of the World Health Organization* 77 (1999): 789–800.

20. S. van der Geest, "The Illegal Distribution of Western Medicines in Developing Countries," *Medical Anthropology* 6 (1982): 197–219.

21. Y.J.F. Hutin, A. M. Hauri, and G. L. Armstrong, "Use of Injections in Healthcare Settings Worldwide, 2000: Literature Review and Regional Estimates," *British Medical Journal* 327 (2003): 1075.

22. E. Drucker, P. G. Alcabes, and P. A. Marx, "The Injection Century: Massive Unsterile Injections and the Emergence of Human Pathogens," *Lancet* 358 (2001): 1989–1992.

23. R. S. Boneva, T. M. Folks, and L. E. Chapman, "Infectious Disease Issues in Xenotransplantation," *Clinical Microbiology Reviews* 14 (2001): 1–14.

24. J. S. Allan, "The Risk of Using Baboons as Transplant Donors: Exogenous and Endogenous Viruses," *Annals of the New York Academy of Sciences* 862 (1998): 87–99.

25. D. Butler, "Last Chance to Stop and Think on Risks of Xenotransplants," *Nature* 391 (1998): 320–324.

26. D. Yoo and A. Giulivi, "Xenotransplantation and the Potential Risk of Xenogeneic Transmission of Porcine Viruses," *Canadian Journal of Veterinary Research* 64 (2000): 193–203.

27. R. A. Weiss, S. Magre, and Y. Takeuchi, "Infection Hazards of Xenotransplantation," *Journal of Infection* 40 (2000): 21–25.

28. Rosenbloom et al., "Biological and Chemical Agents" (see chap. 3, n. 23).

29. D. Ferber, "Microbes Made to Order," *Science* 303 (2004): 158–161.

30. Zinsser quoted in Karlen, *Man and Microbes*, 25 (see chap. 1, n. 17).

31. Jonathan R. Davis and Joshua Lederberg, eds., *Emerging Infectious Disease from the Global to the Local Perspective: Workshop Summary* (Washington, D.C.: National Academy Press, 2001).

32. E. Zwingle, "Cities," *National Geographic*, November 2002, 70–99.

33. Murphy, "Emerging Zoonoses" (see chap. 1, n. 35).

34. Garrett, *The Coming Plague*, 567 (see chap. 1, n. 4)

35. McMichael, *Human Frontiers*, 301 (see chap. 1, n. 8).

36. S. S. Morse, "Factors in the Emergence of Infectious Diseases," *Emerging Infectious Diseases* 1 (1995): 7–15.

37. Arno Karlen, *Biography of a Germ* (New York: Knopf, 2001), 138.

38. A. G. Barbour and D. Fish, "The Biological and Social Phenomenon of Lyme Disease," *Science* 260 (1993): 1610–1616.

39. A. C. Revkin, "Out of Control, Deer Send Ecosystem into Chaos," *New York Times*, November 12, 2002.

40. "Lyme Disease: United States, 2000," *Morbidity and Mortality Weekly Report* 51 (2002): 29–31.

41. A. C. Steere, "Lyme Disease," *New England Journal of Medicine* 345 (2001): 115–125.

42. Taylor et al., "Risk Factors" (see chap. 1, n. 29)

43. P. Saikku, M. Leinonen, K. Mattila et al., "Serological Evidence of an Association of a Novel Chlamydia, TWAR, with Chronic Coronary Heart Disease and Acute Myocar-

dial Infarction," *Lancet* 2 (1988): 983–986; W. H. Frishman and A. Ismail, "Role of Infection in Atherosclerosis and Coronary Artery Disease: A New Therapeutic Target?" *Cardiology in Review* 10 (2002): 199–210; J. B. Muhlestein, E. H. Hammond, J. F. Carlquist et al., "Increased Incidence of *Chlamydia* Species within the Coronary Arteries of Patients with Symptomatic Atherosclerotic versus Other Forms of Cardiovascular Disease," *Journal of the American College of Cardiology* 27 (1996): 1555–1561.

44. C. Storey, M. Lusher, P. Yates et al., "Evidence for *Chlamydia pneumoniae* of Non-human Origin," *Journal of General Microbiology* 139 (1993): 2621–2626; B. Pettersson, A. Andersson, T. Leitner et al., "Evolutionary Relationships among Members of the Genus *Chlamydia* Based on 16S Ribosomal DNA Analysis," *Journal of Bacteriology* 179 (1997): 4195–4205.

45. D. M. Vail and E. G. MacEwen, "Spontaneously Occurring Tumors of Companion Animals as Models for Human Cancer," *Cancer Investigation* 18 (2000): 781–792.

46. H. zur Hausen, "Proliferation-Inducing Viruses in Non-permissive Systems as Possible Causes of Human Cancers," *Lancet* 357 (2001): 381–384; H. H. Skinner, E. H. Knight, and M. C. Lancaster, "Lymphomas Associated with a Tolerant Lymphocytic Choriomeningitis Virus Infection in Mice," *Laboratory Animals* 14 (1980): 117–121.

47. M. V. Viola, "Hematological Malignancies in Patients and Their Pets," *Journal of the American Medical Association* 205 (1968): 95–96.

48. Murphy, "Emerging Zoonoses."

49. Mark S. Smolinski, Margaret A. Hamburg, and Joshua Lederberg, eds., *Microbial Threats to Health: Emergence, Detection, and Response* (Washington, D.C.: National Academy Press, 2003), 245.

50. Smolinski et al., *Microbial Threats to Health*, 165.

51. Ibid., 170.

52. Lederberg et al., *Emerging Infections*, 131 (see chap. 1, n. 36).

53. Tom Burroughs, Stacey Knobler, and Joshua Lederberg, eds., *The Emergence of Zoonotic Diseases* (Washington, D.C.: National Academy Press, 2002), 7.

54. This list is adapted from information in *Animal-Borne Epidemics Out of Control: Threatening the Nation's Health* (Trust for America's Health, 2003), www.healthy americans.org.

55. John Files, "Effort to Coordinate Some Disease Research," *New York Times*, June 3, 2004.

56. Smolinski et al., *Microbial Threats to Health*, 170.

57. L. K. Altman, "As Bird Flu Spreads, Global Health Weaknesses Are Exposed," *New York Times*, February 3, 2004.

58. Smolinski et al., *Microbial Threats to Health*, 170.

59. E. Williamson, "Mad-Cow Fear Raises Concerns in Md. Death," *Washington Post*, January 11, 2004.

60. http://www.aphis.usda.gov/vs/ncie/pet-info.html, accessed July 15, 2003.

61. P. M. Schantz, D. Meyer, and L. T. Glickman, "Clinical, Serologic, and Epidemiologic Characteristics of Ocular Toxocariasis," *American Journal of Tropical Medicine and Hygiene* 28 (1979): 24–28.

62. Morrison, "Zoonotic Infections from Pets" (see chap. 7, n. 119).

63. D. Robertson, P. J. Irwin, A. J. Lymbery et al., "The Role of Companion Animals in the Emergence of Parasitic Zoonoses," *International Journal of Parasitology* 30 (2000): 1369–1377.

CHAPTER 11. A Four-Footed View of History

1. Cartwright and Biddiss, *Disease and History*, 8.

2. H. Weiss, M.-A. Courty, W. Wetterstrom et al., "The Genesis and Collapse of Third Millennium North Mesopotamian Civilization," *Science* 261 (1993): 995–1004.

3. Ibid.
4. Ibid.
5. Bray, *Armies of Pestilence*, 4.
6. *Encyclopaedia Britannica* (1954), s.v. Xerxes.
7. Karlen, *Man and Microbes*, 59.
8. Eva Panagiotakopulu, "Pharaonic Egypt and the Origins of Plague," *Journal of* Bio-geography 31 (2004): 269–275.
9. Exod. 9:3, 9.9 (RSV).
10. Exodus 12:29–30.
11. Ewald, "Evolution and Ancient Diseases," 117–124.
12. McNeil, *Plagues and People*, 121.
13. Karlen, *Man and Microbes*, 73.
14. McNeil, *Plagues and People*, 146.
15. H. G. Wells, *The Outline of History: Being a Plain History of Life and* Mankind (New York: Macmillan, 1925), 553.
16. McNeil, *Plagues and People*, 130.
17. Bray, *Armies of Pestilence*, 14.
18. Edward Gibbon, *The History of the Decline and Fall of the Roman Empire*, chap.10, sec.3, "FamineandPestilence," http://www.ccel.org/g/gibbon/decline/volume1/chap10.htm, accessed May 17, 2004.
19. Zinsser, *Rats, Lice and History*, 139.
20. Cartwright and Biddiss, *Disease and History*, 11.
21. Gibbon, *History of the Decline and Fall*, chap. 43, sec. 3, "Plague," http://www.ccel.org/g/gibbon/decline/volume2/chap43.htm#plague, accessed May 17, 2004.
22. Chase, *The Barbary Plague*, 33.
23. Bray, *Armies of Pestilence*, 47.
24. Zinsser, *Rats, Lice and History*, 133, 131.
25. Ibid., 128.
26. McNeil, *Plagues and People*, 136.
27. Cartwright and Biddiss, *Disease and History*, 18.
28. McNeil, *Plagues and People*, 136–137.
29. Cartwright and Biddiss, *Disease and History*, 15. Zinsser, Rats, Lice and History, 139.

Glossary of Definitions
Related to Microbes

animals	One of three phyla of complex forms of life, the other two being plants and fungi. There are approximately thirty million animal species, of which mammals constitute less than 0.1 percent.
bacteria	Single cells without a nucleus but able to reproduce themselves, probably the oldest form of life on earth.
commensal	A microbe that lives with an animal but does not cause any disease.
DNA	Deoxyribonucleic acid, a large molecule composed of a string of nucleotides and sugars connected by phosphate bonds shaped in the form of a double helix. DNA contains all of our genetic information. DNA encodes RNA, which then encodes proteins, the building blocks of all of our body structures and functions.
endemic	Prevalent in a particular animal or region.
epidemic	Highly prevalent, widespread, and rapidly increasing.
fungi	A large group of organisms related to plants but without green color. The group includes some members that occasionally cause human diseases such as histoplasmosis.
gene	Long strands of DNA, situated on chromosomes in cells, that determine what proteins a cell will express at any given time. Some viruses use RNA instead of DNA as their genes.
host	The animal that is infected.
humans	A species of hominid primate, officially called *Homo sapiens*. As primates, humans are classified as mammals and thus as animals.
microorganism	Literally, a small organism, usually implying bacteria, viruses, and protozoa. Often shortened to *microbe* and in common parlance referred to as "a germ."
mutation	A rare change in the DNA nucleotide pattern, sometimes producing a change in proteins expressed by the cell. Some mutations result in diseases in individuals who have them.
pathogen	A microbe capable of causing disease.

polymorphism   A variation in the DNA nucleotide pattern that occurs commonly in the human population. Some are associated with individual differences in the ability to fight infections.

protozoa   Single cells with nucleus and mitochondria, thus more complex than bacteria. Types include amoeba, flagellates, ciliates, sporozoa, coccidia, and microsporidia.

reservoir   An animal in which large numbers of microbes may be found, often the source of a microbe's spread to other animals.

RNA   Ribonucleic acid, a large molecule encoded by DNA and similar in structure to DNA but different in some of the building blocks. Encodes proteins and has other regulatory functions.

vector   An organism, usually an insect or arthropod, that carries a microbe from one animal to another, such as fleas, flies, ticks, and mosquitoes, e.g., ticks carry the bacteria that causes Lyme disease from deer to humans.

virulence   The relative strength of a particular microbe. Many viruses, bacteria, and protozoa have different strains, some of which are more virulent than others.

viruses   DNA or RNA surrounded by a protein or lipoprotein coat. Viruses are unable to reproduce themselves unless they get into living cells.

zoonosis   A disease caused by microbes that spreads naturally from other animals to humans.

Appendix

Timeline

2 billion years ago	Bacteria, viruses, and protozoa evolve
1 billion years ago	The first animals evolve
155 million years ago	Mammals evolve
60 million years ago	Primates evolve
6 million years ago	Hominids separate from primates
1.7 million years ago	Hominids migrate out of Africa for the first time
1.0 million years ago	Hominids become meat-eating hunters
130,000 years ago	anatomically modern *Homo sapiens* evolves
100,000 years ago	*Homo sapiens* migrate out of Africa
30,000 years ago	Paleolithic people make drawings of animals in caves in France and Spain
14,000 years ago	Domestication of dogs
11,000 years ago	Domestication of sheep
10,000 years ago	Domestication of goats
8–10,000 years ago	Domestication of pigs and cattle; settlement of the earliest towns
5,000 years ago	Domestication of horses; development of earliest centers of civilization

Index

The notation *6f* refers to Figure 1-1 on page 6; *17–18t* refers to Table 2.1 on pages 17–18

About the Authors

E. Fuller Torrey, M.D., is a psychiatrist in Bethesda, Maryland. He is associate director for Laboratory Research at the Stanley Medical Research Institute, professor of psychiatry at the Uniformed Services University of the Health Sciences, and president of the Treatment Advocacy Center. His research focuses on infectious agents as possible causes of schizophrenia and bipolar disorder. He is the author of eighteen books, including *The Roots of Treason*, which was nominated by the National Book Critics Circle as one of 1983's five best biographies.

Robert H. Yolken, M.D., is a pediatrician and a specialist in infectious diseases in Baltimore, Maryland. He is the director of the Stanley Laboratory of Developmental Neurovirology and the Ted and Vada Stanley Distinguished Professor of Pediatrics at the Johns Hopkins University Medical Center. He has authored over three hundred professional papers and book chapters, is an editor of the *Manual of Clinical Microbiology*, and has received numerous awards for his research on infectious diseases. He owns two cats.